Healthy
# ALKALINE
# DIET GUIDE

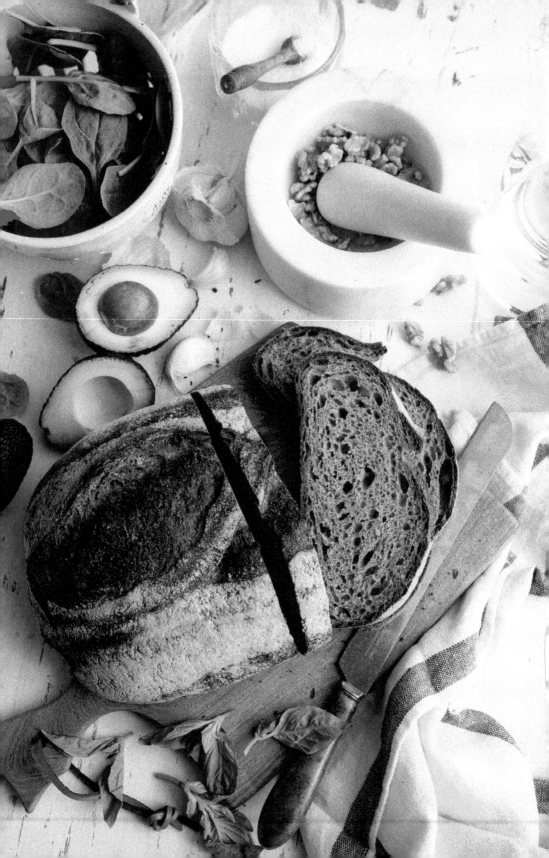

# Healthy
# ALKALINE
# DIET GUIDE

**50** RECIPES / **3**-WEEK MEAL PLAN

## What to Know, Why It Works, and What to Eat

LAUREN O'CONNOR, MS, RDN

Photography by Annie Martin

ROCKRIDGE
PRESS

For general information on our other products and services or to obtain technical support, please contact our Customer Care Department within the United States at (866) 744-2665, or outside the United States at (510) 253-0500.

Rockridge Press publishes its books in a variety of electronic and print formats. Some content that appears in print may not be available in electronic books, and vice versa.

Interior and Cover Designer: Richard Tapp
Art Producer: Meg Baggott
Editor: Justin Hartung
Production Manager: Jose Olivera
Production Editor: Melissa Edeburn

Photography © 2020 Annie Martin. Food styling by Oscar Molinar.
Cover photography by Annie Martin, KarepaStock/Shutterstock, PixelShot/Shutterstock, and DC Studio/Shutterstock.
Author photo courtesy of Violeta Meyners.

ISBN: Print 978-1-64739-348-9 | eBook 978-1-64739-349-6

RO

SAUTÉED EGGPLANT
WITH QUINOA AND
MANGO-CITRUS SALSA
**PAGE 108**

# Contents

# Introduction

If you are reading this book, you are likely someone who thinks about their health. Perhaps you wish to lose weight, you suffer from acne or psoriasis, or you are trying to manage your cholesterol. Regardless, you are here because you want to be healthy.

You may have heard about the alkaline diet from friends, online articles, or even celebrity endorsers. You've also likely heard claims about the diet's benefits, from clearer skin to cancer cures. However, the truth is that the science behind the diet is still being evaluated. Although it is not clearly correlated with all its claimed benefits, the diet is indisputably healthy, in part because it focuses on whole food, plant-based choices.

As a registered dietitian, mother of twins, and resident of Hollywood, California, I've seen many fad diets come and go. I've also taught and witnessed the application of tried-and-true dietary principles that have helped my clients lose weight, reduce their cholesterol, and improve various conditions they had learned to accept until they discovered they had the power to make a difference through healthy lifestyle patterns and sound nutrition.

This book adheres to the belief that no type or amount of food will change your blood's pH because your body has mechanisms in place to naturally regulate pH. As for the diet's other effects on the body, further study and evaluation are warranted. For now, we simply cannot make correlations between the diet and its claims. But by adhering to the dietary principles underscored in this book, you will be eating foods that serve your body best.

I wrote this book for several reasons: First, I want to address and correct the many myths and claims about the alkaline diet. I don't recommend the alkaline diet because of an unproven hypothesis, but rather because it's a whole food, plant-based diet. Second, a healthy alkaline diet can actually benefit you. Third, I want to set you up for success with a foolproof plan for realistic progress and sustainable results.

Let's get started on your journey toward better health.

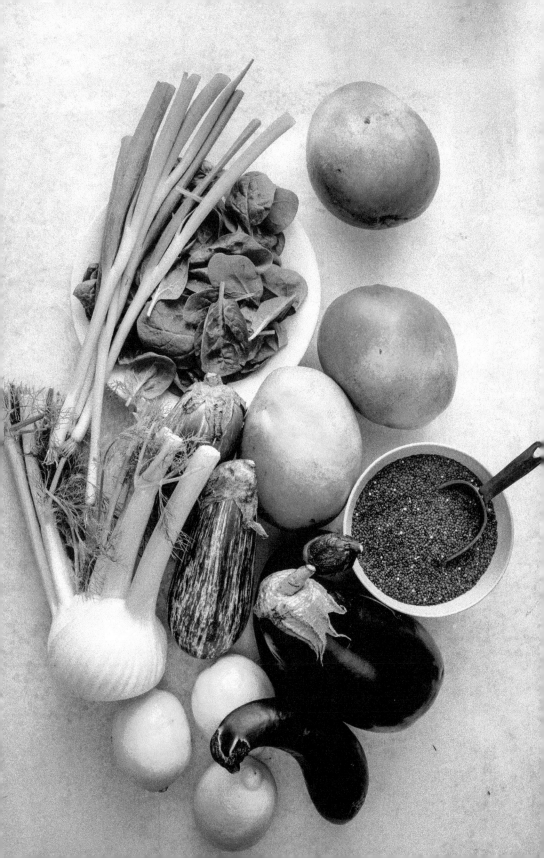

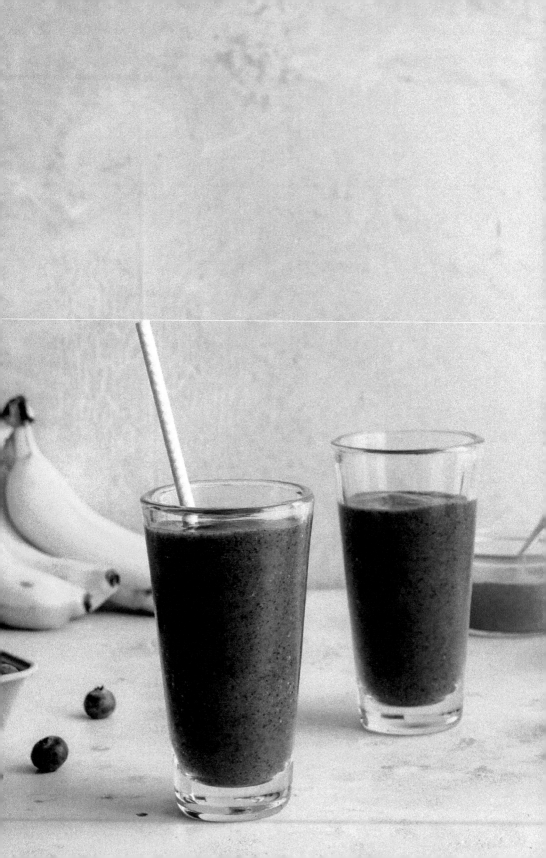

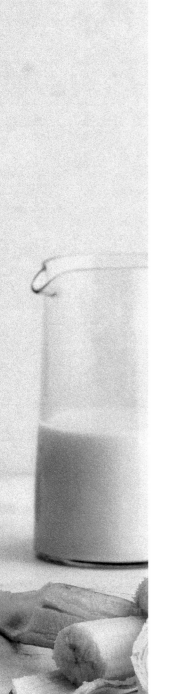

# PART ONE

# Real Talk About the Alkaline Diet

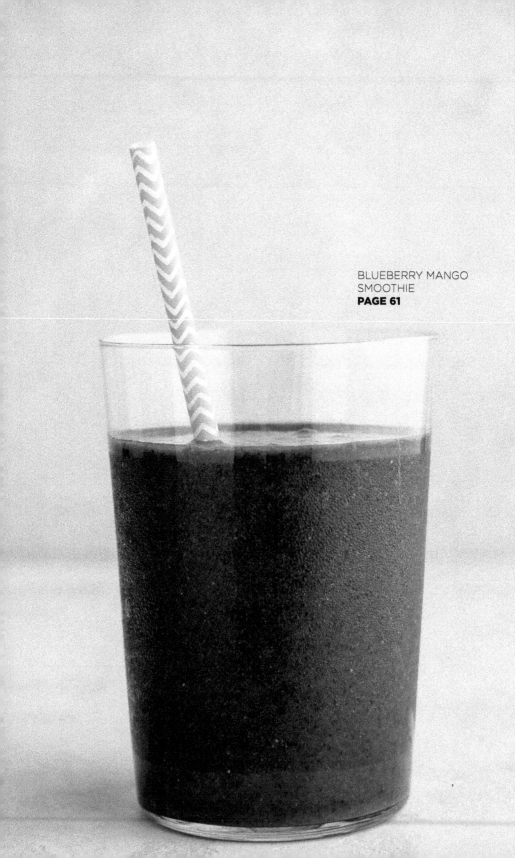

BLUEBERRY MANGO
SMOOTHIE
**PAGE 61**

CHAPTER ONE

# WHAT IS THE ALKALINE DIET?

The alkaline diet is based on the theory that consuming alkaline-promoting foods will directly alter your body's pH to, in effect, treat and prevent disease. Although the alkaline diet encompasses the eating practices of other healthy diets, its primary focus is on the acid-ash hypothesis, which suggests that an acid-forming diet will lead to adverse health consequences, including but not limited to osteoporosis.

The diet follows a plant-based protocol, and science supports limiting red meats, dairy, and highly processed foods in favor of more fruits and vegetables. Adhering to these principles has long been accepted as a sound approach to reducing disease risk and improving quality of life.

To date, there is no conclusive scientific evidence that the alkaline diet works because of the principles on which it was founded. However, it's an indisputably healthy diet option because it focuses on high-quality, nutrient-dense foods. This chapter discusses the basics of the alkaline diet and its health claims—what you need to know, what works, and how this diet can benefit you.

# Alkaline Diet 101

The alkaline diet is a whole food, plant-based, dairy-free diet that encourages eating primarily alkaline-producing foods. The backbone of the diet is based on the acid-ash hypothesis. Supporters of the diet advocate limiting or eliminating meat and dairy because of their acidity, specifically the acid ash they leave behind. They theorize that alkaline-producing foods positively affect your blood pH, and that this in turn elicits health benefits.

Celebrities such as Jennifer Aniston, Victoria Beckham, and Kate Hudson have popularized the alkaline diet. It has also been widely covered in popular health and fitness culture, especially among naturopaths, other alternative health professionals, and their followers. Google searches reached 400,000, and 4.1 million hits for "alkaline diet" and "acid ash diet" respectively, according to an April 2011 review in *Nutrition Journal*.

Like Paleo, Whole30, and other popular diets, the alkaline diet has a specific protocol that should be followed to achieve optimal results. It is key to embrace whole food nutrition and restrict highly processed foods, caffeine, sugar, and alcohol. These simple carbohydrates are the same ones that stimulate your appetite, so limiting them can help you eat less.

Although the Paleo, Whole30, and alkaline diets all focus on eating whole, natural, unprocessed foods, each one allows and restricts particular foods. For example, the alkaline diet includes little, if any, animal protein because it is considered acidic and leaves an acid-ash residue in the body.

The alkaline diet is a food-specific diet, and not designed to be macro-influenced. Restricting certain grains, legumes, and highly processed foods, however, can make this diet low in carbohydrates. Certain fruits or vegetables are limited because of their ash profile, or the pH of the ash left behind once food has been metabolized in the body, rather than their carbohydrate content.

With its whole food, plant-based approach, the alkaline diet can have many benefits (despite its unproven pH promise). The nutrients derived from plant foods benefit the body in many ways, including supporting eye health, skin health, and brain health. Eating more plant foods while limiting red meats, alcohol, sugar, and highly processed foods is a common thread among dietary protocols that have long-standing evidence in promoting positive health outcomes.

# The Science of pH

The measurement that determines the level of acidity or alkalinity in your body is known as pH. On a scale of 1 to 14, 1 is the most acidic and 14 is highly alkaline. A pH of 7 is considered neutral. Various mechanisms regulate the pH in our blood naturally to support our bodies' needs.

## Alkaline

Alkaline refers to a pH range of 8 through 14, with 14 indicating high alkalinity. In the body, pancreatic fluids and compounds such as bone carry alkaline elements, including bicarbonates and calcium. This book considers the alkaline ash foods leave in the body, rather than the pH of these foods in their natural state. Most fruits and vegetables are more alkaline, with some exceptions based on their PRAL score (see the sidebar on page 7).

Foods in the alkaline spectrum include blueberries, beets, asparagus, sweet potato, kale, spinach, and cauliflower. These colorful fruits and vegetables provide a variety of nutrients and antioxidant potential.

## Acid

Acid refers to foods and compounds that retain a pH of 0 through 6. A pH of 7 is considered neutral, and a pH below 3 is highly acidic. Most foods with a low pH leave behind an acid ash indicating that they are acid-forming foods. Animal proteins and dairy are highly acidic.

Acid-forming foods include beef, pork, chicken, cheese, refined sugars, and highly processed foods, including wheat flour, breads, pastas, and cereals. Although most plant foods aren't highly acidic, certain fruits (such as plums and pomegranates) and whole grains (such as buckwheat and brown rice) hit the low-medium acid spectrum. Lemon juice, with a pH of 2 to 3 (acidic in nature), is actually considered alkaline-forming based on the alkaline ash it leaves behind.

# How pH Functions in the Body

What we eat gets converted to energy in a process called metabolism. One of the by-products of this process is an ash residue. This residue is either acidic (pH less than 7) or alkaline (pH greater than 7). The acid-ash hypothesis asserts that diets high in acid-producing foods (those that leave an acid ash) encourage the body to break down bone, leading to osteoporosis. In actuality, bone loss attributable to this mechanism is too minimal to cause osteoporosis.

Regardless of what you eat or the ash that is left behind, your body automatically regulates the pH in your blood. And pH varies in different parts of your body. Despite increases of acid-ash production, high protein intake will not affect the blood's pH, but it can alter the pH of your urine. It's also important to note that the pH of your skin will be different from that of your stomach and saliva.

There are good reasons pH varies in the body. In the skin, natural pH is between 4 and 6.5; this level serves as a barrier to protect it from harmful microbes. In the stomach, pH remains quite low, from 1.3 to 3.5 (an acidic value), to aid in digestion and prevent the overgrowth of certain bacteria. Pancreatic fluid, on the other hand, has a pH of 8.8 (alkaline) in order to neutralize stomach acid, as well as aid in the digestive process.

Thanks to your lungs and kidneys, your body has mechanisms to regulate pH. During the metabolic process, your body breaks down food for effective nutrient delivery, and amino acids are restructured into various proteins to serve your body's needs. As a result of these metabolic breakdown and buildup processes, by-products, including wastes, are formed. The lungs expel this as carbon dioxide, helping to neutralize acidity. The kidneys help by releasing both acids and bases (alkalines) into the bloodstream. Excreting acids in the urine is another way the body maintains its own acid-alkaline homeostasis. A healthy body is thus able to maintain a blood pH of 7.35 to 7.45, independent of the pH of the ash residue of the foods you consume.

The next chapter reviews the acidity and alkalinity of various foods, and there is also a chart starting on page 125.

## IS FOOD ASH A REAL THING?

Food ash is the by-product of a metabolic process that is both catabolic and anabolic in nature, meaning the cycle not only breaks down elements but also produces (or builds) compounds as part of the living process. Food ash is considered an end product; its acidity or alkalinity can be noted in urine. However, contrary to the acid-ash hypothesis, the ash left behind does not affect the pH balance in your blood.

Potential renal acid load (PRAL) scores are used to determine the extent of acid load a food may leave in the body after it is ingested. A food with a positive PRAL score is considered to be acid-producing, and a negative PRAL score indicates a food that is more alkaline or less impacting in the body. Generally, fruits and vegetables are more alkaline, while meats, dairy, and even whole grains and certain beans and legumes are acidic-forming. PRAL is independent of a food's pH value in nature (although they can align in many cases). A lemon, for example, has a natural pH of 1 to 3, but its PRAL score is actually negative, meaning it is alkaline-forming.

# How the Diet Can Actually Help

In this next section, I present the science related to the purported benefits of the alkaline diet: the truths, the fallacies, and the misconceptions. Because this plant-based diet is healthy overall, many of the following conditions may be improved, although not necessarily for the reasons you'd expect.

## Blood Pressure

Cross-sectional, observational studies suggest a potential relationship between dietary acid load and blood pressure. But does this mean an alkaline diet is necessary to keep blood pressure levels in check?

The DASH (Dietary Approaches to Stop Hypertension) diet and similar plant-based diets are rich in potassium and contain plenty of foods with base-producing (alkaline) properties. DASH has been considered an effective means of reducing high blood pressure. Increases in fruit and vegetable consumption, independent of reducing salt and alcohol, have blood pressure–reducing effects.

There is significant, substantial scientific evidence that potassium (a mineral highly present in fruits and vegetables) not only helps maintain sodium balance, but also has a vasodilation effect, which is ideal for overall blood pressure control.

Dietary fiber is also significantly higher in those who follow plant-based diets. Getting plenty of fiber is recommended in DASH and other nutritional interventions as an effective way to treat high blood pressure. Fiber is widely available in fruits, vegetables, whole grains, and legumes.

Despite the alkalinity in most fruits and vegetables, science does not support their alkaline-forming qualities as a measure for blood pressure control.

### The Bottom Line:

Whole food, plant-based diets provide significant benefits for blood pressure control. Furthermore, potassium intake and dietary acid load tend to be inversely related, as higher potassium intakes and lower PRAL scores are indicative of DASH and other healthy plant-based diets. As evidenced by science, potassium, not the alkaline ash of the food, is a key factor.

# Cancer

Cancer thrives in an acidic environment. Some reviews suggest that the disease alters the acid-base homeostasis in the body and tumor cells inhibit the processes the body undergoes to correct adverse imbalances. Can an alkaline diet help correct these imbalances?

Although in vitro and animal studies show that buffer therapy (using oral agents such as bicarbonates to raise tumor pH) might be useful in cancer treatment, this has not been evaluated in human health. To date, there have been no credible systematic reviews to determine that alkaline water or the practice of eating a diet high in alkaline-producing foods will have a direct role in the treatment of cancer.

The American Institute of Cancer Research (AICR) contends that food choices do not affect the body's acidity. Rather, food can influence the nutritional balance necessary in treating and preventing cancer and other life-threatening diseases.

Based on consistent, conclusive evidence, the AICR recommends eating a diet rich in legumes, fruits, vegetables, and whole grains, and limiting consumption of red meat, fast foods, and other processed foods high in starch, fat, and sugar.

### The Bottom Line:

The alkaline diet recommends consuming mainly fruits and vegetables as part of an established pattern shown to prevent cancer. These foods are rich in vitamins, minerals, antioxidants, nutrients, and fiber, all of which support cancer prevention and treatment.

## Bone Health

According to the acid-ash hypothesis, high protein intake is detrimental to bone health because the body robs bone of its minerals in an attempt to neutralize excess acidity. The concern is skeletal bone loss that may be evidenced through increased urinary calcium loss; thus, supporters believe an alkaline diet may be bone-protective.

### Science Says:

Osteoporosis tends to be gradual in effect, and more consistent with aging. The magnitude of acidity in the modern diet would be more than enough to produce a whopping 50 percent bone loss in just 20 years—a rapid progression of osteoporosis, according to a 2008 meta-analysis published in the *American Journal of Clinical Nutrition*. Furthermore, the researchers state, osteoporosis is not measured by urinary calcium loss, but rather by fractures and bone biopsies.

Abnormalities in mineral balance, as well as vitamin deficiencies, may be more likely correlated with bone disease. Phosphorus is essential for bone health and other biological processes. However, excess phosphorus has been associated with adverse effects in the body, including cardiovascular disease and bone disease in those with chronic kidney disease, according to a September 2013 article published in *Advanced Nutrition*.

Science supports that vitamin D deficiency contributes to bone loss because of its connection with magnesium and phosphorus in the mechanisms that support healthy bones. Most people exhibit vitamin D deficiency as they age, which might more likely explain bone deterioration of any extent. Aging is a widely known contributor to osteoporosis.

The National Osteoporosis Foundation suggests fruits and vegetables as supportive of bone health, along with adequate calcium and vitamin D. Additionally, lifestyle factors such as adequate sunlight and regular physical activity, including weight-bearing exercise, may be useful in promoting good bone health. The National Institutes of Health recommends refraining from smoking, and a landmark study showed that smoking increases fracture risk, especially with age.

### The Bottom Line:

The alkaline diet has its merits in supporting overall health, including bone health, with nutrient-dense whole food nutrition via a plant-based diet. Although many people seek calcium from dairy products, which are acid-producing, it can also be obtained via plant foods.

# Weight Loss

Supporters of the alkaline diet believe alkalizing the body will help you drop pounds. They assert that an excess of acid-producing foods creates an acidic environment in which the body produces and holds on to excess fat, and, therefore, that consuming a diet high in alkaline-producing foods purportedly affects pH levels for desired fat loss.

## Science Says:

The kidneys and lungs maintain a tightly regulated pH window of 7.35 to 7.45 in the body. No amount of fruits and vegetables (although many are highly alkaline) will change your blood's pH status. Furthermore, the body mitigates excess acidity by various processes that maintain an acid-base balance through homeostasis.

A Western diet pattern that is high in excess fat and calories, in addition to acid load, contributes to weight gain, obesity, and metabolic disease. Higher acid loads have been associated with higher triglyceride levels, according to a 2019 meta-analysis published in *PLOS ONE*.

There is evidence that lowering processed carbohydrate foods, excess sugars, animal protein, and saturated fats reduces the acid load in one's diet. But a relatively healthy body manages to maintain acid-base balance regardless of diet.

Food cannot affect the pH in the blood. Food choices can have a direct effect on the gut microbiome, however. Research has shown that food can alter the composition of gut bacteria in less than 24 hours. Dietary fiber (more widely available in plant-based diets) can influence gut bacteria composition and has been shown to have favorable effects on health, including blood sugar balance and weight control.

## The Bottom Line:

We know that diets rich in fruits and vegetables and low in saturated fats, animal proteins, and highly processed foods are beneficial to overall health and weight maintenance. These diets are lower in calories and have the benefit of higher dietary fiber, as opposed to diets that include animal proteins and dairy. Switching to a plant-based diet has weight loss benefits unrelated to the pH and acid load of foods ingested. Thus, a healthy alkaline diet can have weight loss benefits, but not necessarily because of its attempts to lower the acid load in the body.

# Pancreatic Health

Pancreatitis is a digestive disorder marked by inflammation and malabsorption of nutrients in the digestive tract, resulting in pain, bloating, nausea, or vomiting. Can an alkaline diet resolve digestive balance and ultimately reduce inflammation?

## Science Says:

A chronic excess of acidity in the body can lower the pH of pancreatic fluids, causing premature activation of digestive enzymes within the pancreas. This causes self-destruction of the pancreas's own tissue, inflammation, and an inability to release digestive enzymes for proper absorption of nutrients. Acute pancreatitis can range from a benign disorder to a life-threatening disease. According to a 2014 review article in *Journal of the Pancreas*, the pancreas is one of the organs most susceptible to damage from a highly acidic environment.

It was previously thought that bowel rest (i.e., fasting) was important to prevent further consequences of the disease. However, current medical nutritional therapy for acute pancreatitis includes an oral soft food diet as tolerated or tube-feeding. Diet therapy is based more on nutrient value (and preventing deficiencies) than the restriction of acid-forming foods.

## The Bottom Line:

Inflammation in the gut is implicated in various digestive issues that may impact our health. Research is still ongoing regarding the direct effects food and diet can have on treating inflammatory diseases. For now, the focus is on intake of nutrient-dense foods.

# Kidney Health

Kidney disease is an inflammatory disorder that centers on the body's inability to properly excrete waste, which leads to excess acidity in the body. Can an alkaline diet reduce excess acidity implicit in kidney disorders and the progression of the disease?

According to multiple, large-cohort analyses, metabolic acidosis is both a cause and effect of chronic kidney disease progression. In patients with kidney disease, the methods the body undergoes to achieve its acid-base balance heavily tax the body, particularly the bones.

The body maintains its acid-base balance through complex mechanisms, borrowing from muscle and bone to obtain minerals like calcium to help buffer acidity. In theory, this may lead to muscle wasting and osteoporosis. However, this theory is not scientific fact. Furthermore, there is no evidence that the pH contribution of a diet can slow the progression or adverse implications of kidney disease.

A more substantial nutritional strategy that helps manage and slow the progression of the disease is a controlled diet (including careful management of protein intake and potassium-rich foods, such as fruits and vegetables), along with drug therapy.

### The Bottom Line:

The alkalinity (or acidity) of a food has no direct effect on acid-base balance in the body. A controlled diet, drug therapy, and dialysis (if necessary) are the current standard of practice for treatment and management of kidney disease.

## Acid Reflux and GERD

Acid reflux is the result of stomach acids flowing back up the esophagus, resulting in heartburn and indigestion. Chronic acid reflux is known as GERD (gastroesophageal reflux disease), and if untreated, it can lead to a condition called Barrett's esophagus, putting one at risk for esophageal cancer. In theory, an alkaline diet can relieve reflux symptoms by eliminating acid-forming foods as a means to prevent indigestion and heartburn.

### Science Says:

Although acidic foods can definitely exacerbate acid reflux, certain foods can loosen the lower esophageal sphincter (LES), making digestive backflow more likely and resulting in symptoms such as heartburn, indigestion, and throat burn. When reflux becomes chronic, the acid backflow can cause damage to the esophagus, throat, and larynx (and even to the sinuses).

Acid-forming foods and alkaline-forming foods are not necessarily defined by their pH value, which determines whether a food is acidic, neutral, or alkaline. The residue, or ash, a particular food may leave in the body is independent of its pH value. A food such as lemon is purported by alkaline-diet supporters to be beneficial because of its alkaline ash, but it can be detrimental to someone who suffers from GERD because of its low pH (acidity), which can irritate and exacerbate already sensitive conditions in the throat and esophagus.

Additionally, alkaline-forming foods such as lemons, limes, oranges, tomatoes, and apple cider vinegar have a natural pH around or below 4 (indicating that they are acidic in nature, despite the alkaline ash they leave behind). Acidic foods activate pepsin, a digestive enzyme in the stomach, which could potentially break down the protective linings of the esophagus and throat in those with GERD.

Dietary recommendations for GERD are based on a whole food, plant-based diet that limits naturally high-pH foods (and any with properties that loosen the LES) in order to reduce exacerbation of symptoms and allow for healing. Digestion of food is also a relevant consideration, as digestive delay (gastroparesis) can trigger excess acid and thus reflux. Foods such as animal meats, cheeses, and saturated fats impact digestion. Digestive delay from rich, high-fat foods can result in fermentation in the stomach and a backflow of acids.

## The Bottom Line:

Reducing naturally acidic foods allows the body to heal. Adhering to a specific food protocol is necessary to reduce the production of excess acid, as well as prevent the aggravation of inflamed tissues. An alkaline diet must be tailored to an acid reflux or GERD treatment regimen to eliminate foods that can cause issues.

# This Book's Approach to the Alkaline Diet

This book's approach to the recipes and overall diet plan is to bring forth the best of the alkaline diet, featuring a plenitude of fruits and vegetables with an emphasis on nutrient-dense whole foods. An 80/20 rule allows for a realistic, accessible, and restriction-free plan.

Whole food, plant-based nutrition from a typical alkaline diet, plus the inclusion of less-alkaline (and perhaps a bit acidic, but still nutritionally beneficial) foods, allows for more nutrient balance. This will help prevent any deficiencies that might result from following a strictly alkaline plan. The healthy alkaline diet presented in this book is essentially a meat-free, dairy-free plan with some wiggle room. The dietary guide provides plenty of protein, calcium, and essential B vitamins from a wealth of plant foods in your diet.

You can definitely benefit from a healthy alkaline diet, even though science doesn't back the pH promise upon which the alkaline diet was founded. As a whole food, plant-based, dairy-free diet, it follows an overall dietary approach that has long been valued and recognized for its role in overall health and disease prevention. Like DASH and the Mediterranean diet, the alkaline plan encourages a high intake of fruits and vegetables, while limiting animal proteins, dairy, and highly processed foods.

I urge you to look at the diet for what it actually brings to the table: a variety of fruits and vegetables, legumes, and intact whole grains—all of which contain a wide range of essential nutrients, including protein-building amino acids and antioxidant compounds to support nutrition and overall health. Ultimately, it is your personal health that is the best indication that the diet is working.

SWEET POTATO AND
CARROT MEDALLIONS
**PAGE 76**

# CHAPTER TWO

# EATING ALKALINE

Eating alkaline means you will be consuming plenty of fruits and vegetables, but it doesn't mean you will be entirely eliminating everything on the acidic spectrum, which includes (surprise!) certain whole grains and legumes that can be highly beneficial to your health and well-being.

This chapter provides insight into which foods are the best options and which foods you should generally limit or avoid; it's essentially a shopping list for the utmost success. We also debunk some current myths about the alkaline diet. This chapter prepares you for the next stage of your journey, including getting your pantry ready, shopping for ingredients, and planning your first month of the alkaline diet using a carefully devised meal plan for optimal nutrition.

# Foods to Eat

For the most part, fruits and vegetables are considered alkaline, while meat, dairy, and highly processed foods are viewed to be more acid-forming.

The concern among supporters of the acid-ash hypothesis is that high levels of acid ash in the body overtax the body's acid-base regulatory mechanisms, which disrupts other regulatory functions in the body. That being said, there remains no scientific validity supporting the notion that you can actually affect your blood pH through consuming alkaline-rich foods. Furthermore, your body may be more capable of regulating blood pH than you think.

We may not entirely understand the etiology in which highly inflammatory conditions, such as kidney disease, develop and progress. But as we learned in the last chapter, implementing a diet rich in plant foods and limited in animal proteins, dairy, and unprocessed foods can shape a healthier outlook for a relatively healthy individual. Alkaline foods are good for your health, primarily because they are plant foods. Plant foods contain a wide variety of essential vitamins, minerals, amino acids, and antioxidants. In their whole form, they provide a synergy of nutritional benefits. Let's take a look at some.

## Dark Leafy Greens

Dark leafy greens include kale, spinach, chard, arugula, and green-leaf and romaine lettuce. They deliver an array of nutrients including vitamins A, C, and K, folate, fiber, magnesium, calcium, iron, and potassium.

## Non-Starchy Vegetables

Non-starchy vegetables include radishes, mushrooms, artichokes, asparagus, broccoli, cauliflower, cucumber, carrots, jicama, peppers, and, of course, leafy greens. They come in a variety of colors and textures, and like leafy greens, they provide very few calories per gram of weight.

# Fruits

When we consider fruits, we are looking at plant foods that not only provide a naturally sweeter taste, but also contain a variety of antioxidant nutrients and essential vitamins and minerals. Fruits are delicious on their own, paired with nuts or nut butters, in salads and healthy green smoothies, and even added as natural sweeteners to balance out flavors in bitter greens like arugula and some savory dishes like curries.

# Nuts

Although nuts are high in calories, they offer healthy monounsaturated and polyunsaturated fatty acids such as omega-3s that are essential for brain function and hormonal regulation in the body. So, include these in your diet, but exercise portion control—1 ounce (2 tablespoons) is considered one serving. Nuts provide nutrients such as magnesium (which helps regulate blood pressure) and immune-supportive vitamin E. According to research, nuts may help lower bad cholesterol, lower levels of inflammation related to heart disease, and improve the structure and lining of your arteries. The American Heart Association suggests consuming 1.5 ounces (3 tablespoons) of unsalted nuts per day, four times per week.

# Seeds

Like nuts, seeds are also calorie-dense but full of nutrients. They also provide polyunsaturated and monounsaturated fats, as well as fiber and nutrients like vitamin E. Consumed in small portions, they can be part of a healthy diet. Like nuts, seeds may help regulate blood sugar (as they are low in carbohydrates and include dietary fiber) and blood pressure. Top your salads or soups with a light sprinkling of seeds to provide a delicate crunch, a bit of flavor, and some added nutrients to your plate.

# Olive Oil and Avocado Oil

These oils are included in your healthy fats because they can help provide you with the essential fatty acids you need. The monounsaturated and polyunsaturated fats in these healthy oils benefit the brain, nerves, skin, nails, and hormonal regulation, too! Used sparingly to lightly coat leafy greens (and when used in combination with spices and other foods), they help carry and distribute flavor to your palate.

## Beans and Other Legumes

These plant foods are special because they are not only rich in complex carbohydrates, but also good sources of protein, making them a part of two food groups. Additionally, they are rich sources of fiber and essential B vitamins.

## Whole Grains

Intact whole grains such as quinoa, buckwheat, and brown rice provide some protein, as well as the benefit of complex carbohydrates, and their fiber content ultimately assists in blood sugar control. They bring B vitamins to the table, as well as a variety of other heart-healthy nutrients, including iron, magnesium, and phosphorus.

## Tofu and Soybeans

Soybeans (known as edamame in their whole, cooked form) can be processed into tofu, which, like its base component, is a good protein source. Yes, tofu is processed, but not highly processed, and thus it doesn't contain a lot of additives. Generally, it is made up of three ingredients: soybeans, water, and a coagulant. Tofu offers the benefit of a convenient source of protein that can easily translate into many different dishes due to the variety of textures available and its mild flavor.

## Apple Cider Vinegar

This vinegar is highly touted in many popularized versions of the alkaline diet. The benefit of this tangy acid (which, like lemon, leaves an alkaline ash in the body) is that its flavor is so intense, just a little can add a lot of flavor to your food. As a fermented food, it may help support digestive health.

# Foods to Avoid

Although this diet is not highly restrictive, there is a very good reason to limit or avoid certain foods. Many of the following foods are not only more acidic, they are also more inflammatory, especially if consumed in large amounts. Even though some of the foods on this list provide some nutritional benefit (e.g., meat is a protein-rich food that contains the essential vitamin $B_{12}$), it is best to focus more on your fruits, veggies, intact whole grains, beans, and legumes. Below are some reasons, beyond their acidity, to limit or avoid the following foods.

## Red Meat

Red meat contains phosphorus, an essential nutrient you can also obtain from plant foods. It is also a very good source of protein and vitamin $B_{12}$. However, it is higher in saturated fat than other proteins, such as chicken, fish, and vegetable proteins. Saturated fats have been correlated with cardiovascular disease risk factors. There is strong evidence that consuming red meat and processed meats causes cancer, particularly colorectal cancer, according to the American Institute for Cancer Research, and a large body of scientific evidence links the high intake of red meat and processed meats to greater risks of heart disease, cancer, and diabetes, according to Harvard Health.

## Processed Meats

Processed meats include sausages, ham, corned beef, smoked meats, and dried meats, which are preserved through curing, salting, smoking, or drying. High intake of processed meats has been implicated in chronic disease, including high blood pressure, cancer, and heart disease.

## Added Sugars

Added sugars include, but are not limited to, refined white sugar, brown sugar, corn syrup, rice syrup, dextrose, honey, malt sugar, and molasses—many of which are found in highly processed foods. Diets high in added sugars are widely known to promote insulin resistance and weight gain. Scientific evidence also reveals that high sugar intake can increase cardiovascular risk, including raising

triglycerides and LDL ("bad") cholesterol and promoting inflammation, blood platelet disruption, and oxidative stress that contributes
to atherosclerosis (hardening of the arteries).

## Dairy

Dairy includes milk, yogurt, kefir, butter, and any of those foods
processed from the milk of an animal (e.g., cow and goat milk). Many
dairy foods have the benefit of containing calcium and protein, and
some, such as yogurt and kefir, contain probiotics. Dairy can con-
tribute to allergies or sensitivities in certain individuals, and some
science supports that it can be inflammatory in the body (although
there is conflicting evidence on this matter). Regardless, limiting
dairy is not detrimental, as you can get plenty of calcium and protein
from a wide variety of plant foods.

## Highly Processed Grains

Highly processed grains include breads, muffins, crackers, tortillas,
cakes, and pastries. The processing of wheat, rice, and other whole
grains into flour (an ingredient in these foods) removes the outer
fiber-rich layer and nutrient-dense germ, leaving behind the starch,
which is rapidly converted to sugar in the body—a process that
can adversely affect blood sugar. Furthermore, highly processed
foods contain additives, including sugars, sodium, chemicals,
stabilizers, and more, that have little benefit for the body, and some
of these (like BHT added as a preservative) are considered toxic.
Additionally, some unexpired, highly processed foods may contain
trans fats if they were manufactured before 2018, when the fats
were banned.

## Alcohol

Wine, beer, vodka, and gin are broad examples of alcohol people may
enjoy. Studies implicate excessive alcohol intake with blood pressure
and heart disease risk. Furthermore, many alcoholic drinks include
added sugars or syrups—further increasing the sugar content of
the drink.

# Coffee

Caffeine may be beneficial for its immediate energy boost, but these effects don't last long. Studies that support its health contributions (as well as deficits to optimal health) are conflicting. Dependency on caffeine can reduce intake of nutrient-dense options if you use it constantly to boost your energy to get through the day.

# Chocolate

When we refer to chocolate, we are generally not talking about the cocoa bean itself, but rather the product it gets processed into, whether it's chocolate chips, a chocolate bar, or cocoa powder for hot cocoa. Consuming sugar-free chocolate is not much better; many people feel that artificial sweeteners give you permission to consume more artificially flavored foods with less nutritional value. Not only does the chocolate we eat contain added sugars or sugar substitutes, it's also calorie-dense and contains caffeine.

# Soda

Sodas are often processed with added sugars or sugar substitutes (non-nutritive sweeteners). Sugar substitutes are highly processed and may not have the overall health benefits one might expect, despite containing little to no calories or sugars. Furthermore, sodas don't provide much nutritional value beyond the phosphorus they contain (which actually may be excessive for anyone who overconsumes soda). Additionally, soda is a diuretic and thus dehydrating. Drinking soda to quench thirst is actually counterproductive, as it often replaces necessary recommended water intake.

# Protein Supplements

Protein supplements include blends of vegetable proteins such as pea protein or animal-derived proteins such as whey protein or collagen. It is important to note that many of these powders or blends are highly processed. Although some supplements may contain a convenient source of protein (and perhaps other additional nutrients), they are highly processed and thus exposed to chemicals used in the processing. It is better to get your nutrients from whole foods.

## THE 80/20 APPROACH

This alkaline diet is not limited to highly alkaline foods; rather, it follows an 80/20 rule. This means you can enjoy a wide variety of foods in the alkaline spectrum, while allowing for foods that fall in the acidic range. Enjoying 80 percent alkaline foods and 20 percent acidic foods makes this diet realistic and unrestrictive.

An overly restrictive diet can set you up for failure. Did you know that two out of five people quit a diet after just seven days? Eighty percent fail to remain on a diet for more than a month. Lifestyle changes are more likely to stick when we don't feel any deprivation. Depending on your overall health goal, cheats can include a 5-ounce glass of red wine, a 2½-inch chocolate chip cookie, or even a 3-ounce piece of steak.

Furthermore, some very healthy, nutritious foods such as barley, buckwheat, bulgur wheat, kidney beans, pinto beans, and even heart-healthy omega-3-rich walnuts fall within the acidic range. These foods help you meet your protein needs and fiber requirements, and provide specific nutrients that you might otherwise miss in a restrictive alkaline diet. We wouldn't want you to lose out on the nutritional benefits of these foods.

# 5 Myths About the Alkaline Diet

There are many myths about the alkaline diet. Here are the most common, and the truth behind them.

## You Have to Drink Alkaline Water

You don't have to drink alkaline water. Much of the science that supports this assertion is funded by companies that market this product. As with food, there is no substantial scientific evidence to support that alkaline water or drinks will change your blood pH.

According to a 2016 systematic review published in *BMJ*, despite the promotion of the alkaline diet and alkaline water to support cancer treatment, there is a lack of scientific evidence to substantiate this claim. More than 8,000 citations were identified and over 250 abstracts reviewed for this scientific analysis.

## You Have to Take Supplements

While following the alkaline diet, some people have concerns about getting enough B$_{12}$, calcium, iron, vitamin D, and protein. Fortunately, you can get enough of all these from the following healthy, natural sources:

B$_{12}$: nutritional yeast, fortified soy milk, tofu

Calcium: almonds, broccoli, strawberries, beans, peas, lentils, soybeans, chia seeds, flaxseed

Iron: lentils, chickpeas, tofu, cashews, chia seeds, apricots, kale, raisins, quinoa (combining these iron-rich foods with a source of vitamin C such as oranges or strawberries will improve iron absorption in the body)

Vitamin D: sunlight is a free source of vitamin D (according to research, you only need 10 minutes of sun exposure per day to promote the production of vitamin D in the body); you can also obtain it from mushrooms and fortified plant-based milks

Protein: soy milk, soybeans, beans and legumes, nuts, seeds, and a wide variety of leafy greens and non-starchy vegetables for their varying amino acid compositions

Some supplements can be helpful, but it really depends on individual needs. For example, B$_{12}$ deficiencies are easily masked by high intake of folate (highly present in plant foods). Nutritional yeast fortified with B$_{12}$ is considered a good source for vegans, as 1 tablespoon can provide as much as 5 micrograms of B$_{12}$ (that's approximately twice the RDA for adult men and non-pregnant, non-lactating women). And although sunlight is a free source of vitamin D, some individuals have more susceptibility for inadequate absorption.

Additionally, multivitamin supplementation is beneficial to any individual, especially adults over 50 who are at increased risk of poorer absorption of nutrients from food. Although supplementation isn't a must for everyone who follows a healthy alkaline diet, it can be beneficial.

## You Can't Eat Any Meat or Fish

There are many variations of the alkaline diet, some stricter than others. Most alkaline diets have an 80/20 or 70/30 rule, allowing for some flexibility to include a small percentage of meat or fish. Specific nutrients may be difficult to obtain from a strictly vegan diet. These include $B_{12}$ (which is more actively available in animal sources) and certain forms of omega-3s that are not present in plant foods.

Fatty fish, such as salmon, is recommended, as it is a direct source of eicosapentaenoic acid (EPA), an essential omega-3. Therefore, I'm providing you with some things to consider regarding whether you choose to include these in your healthy alkaline diet.

## It's Dangerous

No particular food or drink can change your blood pH, so you are not at risk for alkalosis by following an alkaline diet. According to the Merck Manual, metabolic alkalosis is a manifestation of extreme fluid and electrolyte losses (i.e., sodium and potassium) that can occur as a result of excessive vomiting, kidney malfunction, overactive adrenals, or diuretics. However, those who place strict emphasis on solely alkaline foods can be at risk for nutrient deficiencies. (This healthy alkaline diet does not promote such exclusivity.) Furthermore, excessive food restriction can lead to unhealthy relationships with food (eating disorders), as well as some symptoms that may occur in anorexic individuals, including amenorrhea (lack of menstrual periods) and risk factors for heart arrhythmia (alarmingly low heart rate and blood pressure).

When it comes to potential nutrient deficiencies, through a well-planned alkaline diet (which is essentially vegan), you can obtain all your essential nutrients. However, depending on the individual, supplementation may be necessary.

## The Alkaline Diet
## Is Just a Weight-Loss Diet

Weight loss may be a desired side effect of the alkaline diet. However, the intent and overall design of this whole food, plant-based diet is to deliver optimal health conditions for disease risk prevention. Limiting red meats, dairy, and highly processed foods in favor of higher intakes of fruits and vegetables usually leads to weight loss because plant foods are lower in calories but high in nutrient density and dietary fiber—all factors that promote blood sugar control, satiety, and, ultimately, weight loss.

### CONSIDERATIONS REGARDING LEAN MEAT AND SEAFOOD INTAKE

Plant foods contain limited amounts of vitamin $B_{12}$ (cobalamin). Furthermore, there is great variability in the amounts from sources that are actually available for our needs. Nutritional yeast fortified with $B_{12}$ is considered a good choice for those who don't eat meat, although including some meat in the diet (as per the 80/20 rule) can be beneficial, specifically for this nutrient. Animal proteins (including fish, meat, and eggs) are considered more plentiful sources of $B_{12}$, according to a 2016 article review published in *Nutrients*.

The 2015–2020 Dietary Guidelines for Americans recommend getting a portion of omega-3 fatty acids from seafood each week, because seafood is a direct source of EPA (an essential omega-3). Plant sources are limited to alpha-linoleic acid (ALA), a form of omega-3 that must be converted to exhibit any biological benefit of EPA. However, much of ALA is oxidized in the body, and only a modest amount can be converted, so the omega-3 benefit from seafood sources is greater, according to an article published in the *Journal of the American Dietetic Association*.

# Should You Test Your pH?

You don't need to be concerned with the pH value of a food once ingested. The alkaline-forming nature of a food doesn't change your tightly controlled blood pH. Neither saliva nor urine can indicate blood pH. So is testing your pH necessary? No.

The normal pH for saliva is between 6.2 and 7.6 (it can change depending on what you eat). According to the American Association for Clinical Chemistry, the average pH of urine is 6.0, but can range from 4.5 to 8.0. Abnormal pH values in urine can indicate issues such as kidney stones, UTIs, or other infections. But if you are having certain pain or abnormal issues that require pH testing, you should see a doctor who will perform a urinalysis anyway to determine your diagnosis and recommended treatment.

Overall, a high-quality, whole food, plant-based diet will produce the health benefits you desire. There is a synergy of nutrients contained within whole plant foods working together to provide the immunity, antioxidant benefits, and anti-inflammatory effects (among the many benefits) for your overall health. And given that you cannot directly alter the chemistry of your blood through the pH aspect of a food, I don't believe testing your pH is necessary if you are relatively healthy.

However, for those of you who are curious and wish to test your pH, here is a simple method for doing so.

1. **Obtain pH test paper.** You can get a pH test kit such as MedLab Diagnostics from Amazon. The kit will test the acidity or alkalinity of your saliva or urine. A number at the high end (above 7) indicates more alkaline, and lower numbers (below 7) indicate acidity.

2. **Upon waking, test your urine or saliva.** Follow the instructions on the box. Essentially, you take a pH test strip and dip it into a small sample cup of your saliva or urine. The strip will turn a certain color. Use the chart provided on the back of the test kit to find the corresponding number, which will indicate the level of acidity or alkalinity of your urine.

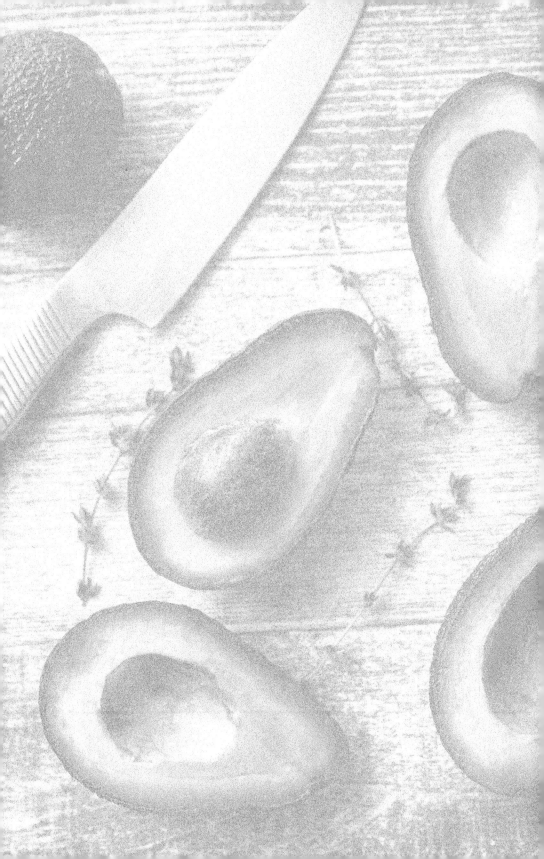

ROASTED CARROT-
TOMATO SOUP
**PAGE 94**

# CHAPTER THREE

# PREPARING FOR THE 21-DAY PLAN

Now that you know the essential foods for this plan, it's time to set up your kitchen. This chapter covers refrigerator and pantry staples, recommends kitchen equipment, and provides a simple three-week meal plan using heart-healthy recipes from this book. This handy guide will get you started with confidence.

You'll have everything in place to make your transition toward healthier eating as smooth and convenient as possible. Many of the recipes rely on certain staples that you will use over and over again, so keep these in stock. This chapter also includes tips to help you stay on course, including how to curb your cravings and what to do if you fall off the wagon. Let's get started.

# Kitchen Prep

Your first step is to set up your kitchen for healthy eating. You'll have to do a bit of a reset to start fresh. It's worth it, however: Not only is it easier to work in a kitchen that has everything you need at hand or within reasonable reach, it also helps keep things organized. Knowing your way around the kitchen and what tools work best can speed up your prep time and keep things simple.

You'll remove or limit foods that don't serve you best, and make more space for what's essential to the diet. Your kitchen will have a fresh appeal that will make your journey new and exciting.

## Tips for Resetting

In a perfect world, you wouldn't be distracted from your focus on your health. But you won't be living in a bubble that shields you from temptation. It is important to start this journey knowing you can get past any obstacles, although it is helpful to have the support of those closest to you.

Although it would be great to get the whole family on board, this may not be possible. It is important to have a discussion with your whole family before you begin your journey. Let them know the health benefits you are seeking and the important reasons behind improving your health (e.g., more energy, getting in better shape to stay active with your kids). Explain that this is not a temporary transition but rather a steady path toward an overall healthy lifestyle. This conversation also applies to your friends and to relatives who aren't living with you.

You and your family will find that healthy eating can be tasty, enjoyable, and satisfying. But don't expect everyone to jump in right away. Stay in control by learning to navigate through challenges that come your way. You can designate your own personal shelf in the refrigerator, or set up a separate area for those still eating snack foods not in your best interest. Make it as easy as possible to grab the foods that will nourish and serve you.

## Refrigerator and Pantry Essentials

Here are some inexpensive, widely available foods to stock in your' refrigerator, freezer, and pantry to get you started on the alkaline diet.

## Refrigerator

- Almond meal
- Broccoli
- Carrots, shredded
- Chia seeds
- Coconut flakes, fine, unsweetened
- Flax meal
- Salad greens
- Tofu

## Freezer

- Bananas (peeled, halved, and stored in resealable baggies)
- Edamame
- Green beans
- Mango chunks
- Petite peas
- Raspberries
- Wild blueberries

## Pantry

**SPICES**

- Cinnamon, ground
- Cumin, ground
- Garlic powder
- Nutritional yeast
- Sea salt
- Thyme, dried

## OIL

- ○ Avocado oil
- ○ Olive oil

## WHOLE GRAINS, FLOUR, AND BAKING SUPPLIES

- ○ Baking powder
- ○ Baking soda
- ○ Brown rice
- ○ Brown rice flour, or your favorite gluten-free flour blend (look for a simple blend such as brown rice flour, chickpea flour, and tapioca starch)
- ○ Quinoa
- ○ Rolled oats, gluten-free

## DRIED FRUIT AND NUTS/SEEDS

- ○ Almonds, whole, raw
- ○ Almonds, sliced
- ○ Cashews, raw
- ○ Dates
- ○ Pumpkin seeds, hulled
- ○ Raisins
- ○ Walnuts, raw

## COUNTER

- ○ Apples
- ○ Avocados
- ○ Bananas

- Garlic cloves*
- Ginger, fresh*
- Lemons
- Pears

*Jarred crushed (or frozen cubed) garlic and ginger offer a no-fuss way to season your dishes without peeling, grating, or crushing.

## CANNED FOODS

- Black beans, low-sodium
- Chickpeas, low-sodium
- Lentils, low-sodium
- Tomatoes, low-sodium

If you have even just a bit of counter space, keep fresh fruit available in a highly visible location and in an appealing arrangement. This is to ensure that you (a) eat it before it goes bad, and (b) remember to reach for fruit instead of less healthy snacks.

Keep these fruits on your counter until it's necessary to refrigerate them. For example, it's great to have an avocado fresh and ready to eat, but if it becomes ripe before you have a chance to eat it, simply store it in the refrigerator to slow further ripening. Do the same with softer fruits like pears and bananas.

If you wish to speed the ripening of your avocado, place a banana on top of it. Ripening bananas release a natural plant hormone called ethylene that hastens the ripening of mature fruits such as avocados.

# Basic Kitchen Equipment

Simplicity was one of the key factors in designing the tasty recipes in this book. However, a few affordable pieces of kitchen equipment will help you get the best results.

## High-speed blender

This will be handy for your quick morning or afternoon smoothies. Even a small 2-cup blender will do.

## Food processor

You'll need this to process whole food ingredients for certain batters, like muffins or cookies. Because we aren't using sugars, fruits such as dates will have to be broken down and well incorporated into the mixture of ingredients.

## Coffee grinder

You can use this to grind nuts or seeds or whole grains like oats into flour. (If you have a small, powerful blender, you can use that instead.)

## Can opener

Canned beans are more convenient than dried legumes, and most canned products require a can opener.

## Mixing bowls

You'll need a variety of bowls, as you may have liquid blends and dry blends to prepare separately and then combine. Not every dish requires a huge bowl, so a nesting set is a great idea. It also saves drawer space.

## Measuring cups and measuring spoons

Many of the dishes created for this book rely on specific measurements for flavor and portion control. Be sure to have a set of measuring cups for dry ingredients and a spouted glass measuring cup for liquids.

## Baking dishes and baking pans

You will need a 9-by-13-inch glass baking dish and an 8- or 9-inch square glass baking dish for the recipes in this book, along with a standard 12-cup muffin tin and a nonstick baking sheet.

## Pans and pots (with lids)

The recipes in this book can be made in 6-inch, 8-inch, or 12-inch nonstick skillets. You will also need a 2-quart saucepan and a 6- to 8-quart stockpot.

## Other handy tools

- **Potato masher or whisk**
- **Garlic press**
- **Hand grater**

## TIPS FOR STAYING ON COURSE

### CURB CRAVINGS

Adjusting to a new dietary plan has its challenges, and cravings are one of the biggest. This diet is not overly restrictive, but you may still find yourself challenged by temptations from time to time. Here are some tips for exercising control without feeling deprived:

- **Take a deep breath.** Or count to 10 slowly. This is what I call "hitting the pause button." Give yourself some time to focus on you and not the food. This pause will help prevent impulse eating.

- **Be mindful.** Set the stage for relaxed eating. Chew slowly, enjoy each bite, and be in the moment. When you focus on your food without distraction, you are more likely to find satisfaction.

- **Drink a glass of water.** Sometimes we misinterpret thirst for hunger. If, after drinking a glass of water, you still feel hungry, reach for a healthy snack like a piece of fruit.

## PLAN AHEAD

Planning your meals and snacks ahead of time will prevent you from reaching for unhealthy convenience choices. You might choose a day to prep ahead for the whole week, or maybe you prefer to do it just a day ahead. Do what works best for you. If you need grab-and-go snacks or meals, make sure they are conveniently portioned and well packed. This is important, especially if you will be out of the house for several hours and healthy choices may not be readily available.

Simple meal prep can range from pre-chopping and storing veggies for convenience to making ready-to-eat lunches for the entire week. You may even find it works best for you to have your dinner leftovers over the next two to three days. Just be sure you include plenty of veggie options throughout the day!

## GET EXERCISE

Some of my clients have discovered that exercising gives them more energy. I always say "energy begets energy." So get off the couch and start moving! Exercising not only helps with muscle tone, cardiovascular fitness, and bone health, but also prevents eating out of boredom.

Keep a regular exercise schedule, such as one hour of cardio or a mixture of cardio, weights, and stretching, three to four times per week. This will help you stay on track and be accountable to yourself in your health goals. When we exercise, we are also reminding ourselves that nourishment is important. And when we start to see results, whether through an endorphin high or weight loss, we generally keep up our healthy eating habits, too.

## GET ADEQUATE SLEEP

Burning the candle at both ends may seem effective, especially when you have a project deadline or are juggling work and family. But if you are frequently burning the midnight oil, you are at risk for insufficient sleep, which can derail your progress.

Be sure to plan for eight hours of sleep each night. Adequate sleep prevents excess production of cortisol, which not only makes us hungrier the following day, but also increases our sweet and starchy cravings. It can also impact your exercise schedule because you may feel too tired to get yourself to the gym or go for a brisk walk. Adequate sleep will help you feel refreshed the next day so you can stay motivated in your journey toward better health.

## SPACE MEALS EVENLY THROUGHOUT THE DAY

Eat within an hour of waking, and space out your meals evenly. For some people, this is every three to four hours; for others, it may be every five to six. Consistency will help prevent cravings as well as afternoon binges and late-night snacking.

Healthy snacks between meals (one or more, depending on your needs) can help suppress cravings, too. Just be sure you are eating in response to hunger and not because you are thirsty or bored. Remember, it's always a good idea to hit the pause button if you are not sure. Reach for a glass of water before you take a bite; you may find you weren't as hungry as you thought.

Finally, give yourself enough time to properly digest your food. It's best to wait at least three hours after eating before hitting the sack. This will prevent acid reflux (and those extra calories that accumulate from late-night snacking).

## IF YOU FALL OFF THE WAGON, GET BACK ON

You may have fallen off the wagon a few times in your life. Don't be afraid of a misstep. Put it in perspective—it is just one meal or one day. It doesn't have to become a pattern.

Get back on track as soon as possible. Allow yourself to digest everything before your next meal, and hydrate as needed. Start the next day anew. As long as you get right back on track, you will prevent a spiral of negative habits that can delay your progress.

You are human, and it's okay to make a mistake. One bad meal or one bad day doesn't need to turn into a cycle of unhealthy eating. Don't make it an all-or-nothing proposition—this rarely leads to success. There may be bumps in the road or minor breaks in your plan, but you can keep moving ahead with an outlook toward the bigger picture: building a lifestyle of healthy habits.

## STAY HYDRATED

It's easy to ignore thirst. Often, we don't recognize our need for water unless we've exerted ourselves through exercise or physical labor, or when it's hot outside. Adequate water intake throughout the day helps with digestion and regularity, and can help prevent cravings, too. Aim for eight 8-ounce glasses spaced out over the course of the day. If you start your day with one or two glasses of water, it's easier to keep a daily habit of drinking enough.

If drinking plain water is a challenge, add a few slices of cucumber or thinly sliced fresh fruit with basil or mint to give it some flavor and make it more visually appealing. You may also enjoy sparkling water, as long as you don't suffer from acid reflux issues.

# Meal Plan

Shifting to a new diet is much easier when you have a structure to follow. This 21-day meal plan will give you a pathway to success with a variety of flavors and textures. Strategic use of leftovers, as well as using many of the same ingredients in multiple ways, will shorten your time in the kitchen, cut food waste, simplify your shopping, and save you money. Let this plan inspire you to create your own plans based on this book's guidelines, tools, and recipes.

## DAY ONE

*Breakfast*
Blueberry Mango Smoothie (page 61)

*Lunch*
Mock Egg Salad (page 87)
+1 cup leafy greens with Dijon Vinaigrette (see page 77)

*Dinner*
Seasoned Lentil Tacos with Bell Peppers and Onions (page 106)
+1 cup steamed broccoli

*Snack*
1 medium apple
+7 cashews

## DAY TWO

*Breakfast*
Maple Oat Flax Granola (page 60)

*Lunch*
Black Bean Veggie Tostada (page 102)
+Carrot Fennel Slaw (page 77)

*Dinner*
Roasted Carrot-Tomato Soup (page 94)
+1 cup salad greens with Dijon Vinaigrette (see page 77)

*Snack*
¾ cup chopped mango

# DAY THREE

*Breakfast*
Banana Berry Chia Pudding (page 66)

*Lunch*
Almond-Crusted Tofu (or salmon) with Mango-Citrus
Salsa (page 113)
+1 cup steamed broccoli

*Dinner*
Roasted Carrot-Tomato Soup (page 94)
+8 olives

*Snack*
Carrot Fennel Slaw (page 77)

# DAY FOUR

*Breakfast*
Maple Oat Flax Granola (page 60)

*Lunch*
Quinoa Black Bean Veggie Bowl (page 103)

*Dinner*
Almond-Crusted Tofu (or salmon) with Mango-Citrus
Salsa (page 113)
+Carrot Fennel Slaw (page 77)

*Snack*
1 medium apple
+7 almonds

## DAY FIVE

*Breakfast*
Banana Berry Chia Pudding (page 66)

*Lunch*
Creamy Zucchini Soup (page 91)
+1 slice whole-grain toast with 1 tablespoon peanut butter

*Dinner*
Quinoa Black Bean Veggie Bowl (page 103)

*Snack*
2 Deviled Eggs (page 74)

## DAY SIX

*Breakfast*
Blueberry Mango Smoothie (page 61)

*Lunch*
Vegan Stuffed Eggplant (page 109)

*Dinner*
Creamy Zucchini Soup (page 91)
+1 cup leafy greens with Dijon Vinaigrette (see page 77)

*Snack*
¼ avocado, sliced
+1 small tomato

## DAY SEVEN

*Breakfast*
"Cheesy" Tofu Scramble with Spinach (page 68)

*Lunch*
2 Deviled Eggs (page 74)
+1 cup steamed broccoli
+1 slice whole-grain toast smeared with 1/4 avocado

*Dinner*
Vegan Stuffed Eggplant (page 109)

*Snack*
3/4 cup blueberries
+2 tablespoons sliced almonds

*Dessert*
Baked Apple Crumble (page 117)

## DAY ONE

### *Breakfast*
1 Blueberry Flax Muffin (page 64)
+¹/₂ avocado, sliced

### *Lunch*
Vegan Spinach-Basil Pesto with Pasta (page 100)
+1 cup steamed broccoli

### *Dinner*
Zucchini Frittata with Tofu "Ricotta" and Lemon (page 104)
+1 cup steamed green beans

### *Snack*
³/₄ cup strawberries

## DAY TWO

### *Breakfast*
Mock "Wheat Porridge" (page 62)

### *Lunch*
Zucchini Frittata with Tofu "Ricotta" and Lemon (page 104)

### *Dinner*
Strawberry Spinach Salad (page 90)
¹/₂ cup cooked and shelled edamame

### *Snack*
1 Blueberry Flax Muffin (page 64)

# DAY THREE

*Breakfast*
1 Blueberry Flax Muffin (page 64)
+¾ cup berries

*Lunch*
Seasoned Lentil Tacos with Bell Peppers and Onions (page 106)

*Dinner*
Vegan Spinach-Basil Pesto with Pasta (page 100)
+1 cup leafy greens

*Snack*
Medium apple

# DAY FOUR

*Breakfast*
Carrot Cake Breakfast Porridge (page 58)

*Lunch*
Strawberry Spinach Salad (page 90)
+3 ounces tofu, chopped

*Dinner*
Vegan Cauliflower-and-Mushroom Lasagna (page 112)

*Snack*
Green Beans Almondine (page 72)

WEEK TWO

## DAY FIVE

*Breakfast*
"Cocoa" Almond Smoothie (page 67)

*Lunch*
Vegan Cauliflower-and-Mushroom Lasagna (page 112)

*Dinner*
Curried Carrot and Raisin Tofu Salad (page 86)
served over 1 cup leafy greens

*Snack*
1 cup sliced strawberries
+1 tablespoon sliced almonds

## DAY SIX

*Breakfast*
Mock "Wheat Porridge" (page 62)

*Lunch*
3 ounces tofu, pan-seared in 1 teaspoon oil
+Green Beans Almondine (page 72)

*Dinner*
Creamy Zucchini Soup (page 91)
+2 whole-grain crackers
+4 olives

*Snack*
1 hard-boiled egg with 1 teaspoon mustard
+1/2 cup raw carrots

*Breakfast*
"Cocoa" Almond Smoothie (page 67)

*Lunch*
Strawberry Spinach Salad (page 90)
+½ cup chickpeas

*Dinner*
Vegan Cauliflower-and-Mushroom Lasagna (page 112)

*Snack*
Avocado Toast with Vegan Spinach-Basil Pesto (page 80)

*Dessert*
2 Cashew Date Oat Bites (page 122)

WEEK TWO

## DAY ONE

*Breakfast*
2 Cashew Date Oat Bites (page 122)
+1/2 banana

*Lunch*
Creamy Zucchini Soup (page 91)
+2 whole-grain crackers
+4 olives

*Dinner*
Fennel-Seasoned Falafel with Hummus Dressing (page 110)
+Green Beans Almondine (page 72)

*Snack*
1 cup diced frozen mango

## DAY TWO

*Breakfast*
Banana Berry Chia Pudding (page 66)

*Lunch*
Fennel-Seasoned Falafel with Hummus Dressing (page 110)
+1 cup arugula with 1 to 2 teaspoons oil and a squeeze of lemon juice

*Dinner*
Curried Carrot and Raisin Tofu Salad (page 86)
+1 cup steamed broccoli

*Snack*
Green Beans Almondine (page 72)

# DAY THREE

*Breakfast*
Tropical Overnight Oats (page 63)

*Lunch*
Curried Carrot and Raisin Tofu Salad (page 86)
+1 cup steamed broccoli

*Dinner*
Zucchini and Pesto Grain Bowl (page 111)
+2 ounces tofu, sliced

*Snack*
1 cup frozen mango chunks
+ frozen wild blueberries

# DAY FOUR

*Breakfast*
Banana Berry Chia Pudding (page 66)

*Lunch*
Zucchini and Pesto Grain Bowl (page 111)
+1/2 cup chickpeas

*Dinner*
Sautéed Eggplant with Quinoa and Mango-Citrus Salsa (page 108)

*Snack*
Almond-Stuffed Dates with Coconut (page 73)

## DAY FIVE

*Breakfast*
Tropical Overnight Oats (page 63)

*Lunch*
Vegan Pumpkin Chili (page 107)
+2 whole-grain crackers

*Dinner*
Sweet Pumpkin and Apple Soup (page 92)
+Green Beans Almondine (page 72)

*Snack*
1 cup raw zucchini slices
+2 tablespoons Simple Hummus with Crudités (page 79)

## DAY SIX

*Breakfast*
"Cocoa" Almond Smoothie (page 67)

*Lunch*
Sweet Pumpkin and Apple Soup (page 92)
+1 cup steamed green beans

*Dinner*
Sautéed Eggplant with Quinoa and Mango-Citrus Salsa (page 108)

*Snack*
1 hard-boiled egg
+1 teaspoon Dijon mustard

# DAY SEVEN

### *Breakfast*
Mango Quinoa Breakfast Porridge (page 59)

### *Lunch*
Vegan Pumpkin Chili (page 107)
+1 cup steamed broccoli

### *Dinner*
Chickpea Rainbow Salad (page 97)

### *Snack*
Almond-Stuffed Dates with Coconut (page 73)

### *Dessert*
Blueberry-Banana Soft Serve (page 116)

WEEK THREE

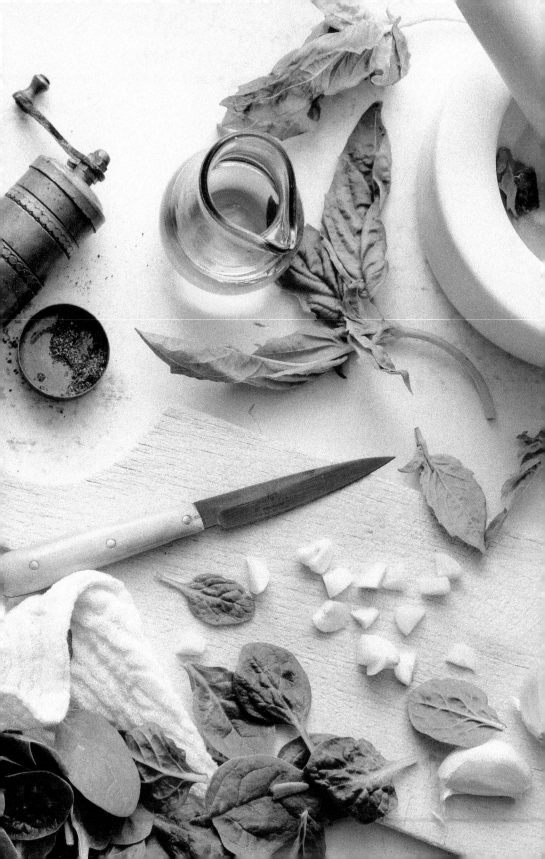

# PART TWO

# The Recipes

TROPICAL OVERNIGHT OATS
**PAGE 63**

# CHAPTER FOUR

# BREAKFASTS AND SMOOTHIES

# Carrot Cake Breakfast Porridge

SERVES 2

**PREP TIME:** 3 minutes / **COOK TIME:** 5 minutes

I created this dish while trying to figure out what to do with my produce at the end of the week. A handful of grapes, some carrots, a ripe banana, and some very handy pantry staples came together to create this delicious porridge.

½ ripe medium banana (save the other half for a same-day snack)

¼ cup red seedless grapes (approximately 12 grapes)

¼ cup shredded carrots

2 small dates, pitted

2 tablespoons unsweetened shredded coconut

⅛ teaspoon ground cinnamon

⅛ teaspoon vanilla extract

½ cup plus 2 tablespoons rolled oats, divided

½ cup unsweetened almond milk

1. In a food processor, combine the banana, grapes, carrots, dates, coconut, cinnamon, vanilla, and 2 tablespoons of oats. Process for 1 to 2 minutes, until well combined.

2. Add the remaining ½ cup of oats and pulse a few times to leave a bit of oat texture.

3. Transfer the mixture to a small saucepan and stir in the almond milk. Heat on medium-low heat for about 5 minutes, until warmed.

**MEAL PREP TIP:** Make a double batch of the breakfast porridge and use the extra batch to make carrot cake muffins. In a large bowl, mix the porridge with ¼ cup avocado oil and 1 medium egg. Stir in ½ cup flax meal, ½ cup all-purpose flour, and 1 tablespoon baking powder. Bake in a preheated 350°F oven for 20 to 25 minutes, until a toothpick inserted into the center of a muffin comes out clean.

**Per Serving (¾ cup):** Calories: 208; Fat: 6g; Protein: 5g; Carbohydrates: 37g; Fiber: 6g; Sodium: 62mg; Iron: 2mg

# Mango Quinoa Breakfast Porridge

SERVES 4

**PREP TIME:** 5 minutes / **COOK TIME:** 25 to 30 minutes

Did you know quinoa has all nine essential amino acids and twice as much fiber as most grains? With a bit of fruit, nut milk, and a little cinnamon, it's a satisfying and nourishing breakfast option.

**3 cups cooked quinoa, cooled**

**1 cup frozen mango chunks, cut into ½-inch cubes**

**¾ cup unsweetened almond milk, plus more for serving**

**¼ teaspoon ground cinnamon**

**⅛ teaspoon sea salt**

1. In an airtight container, mix the quinoa, mango, almond milk, cinnamon, and salt and refrigerate for a couple of hours or up to overnight.

2. Reheat before serving. Add a splash or two of almond milk for the desired consistency.

**LOVING YOUR LEFTOVERS:** Store any remaining porridge in a sealed container in the refrigerator for up to 5 days.

**Per Serving (1 cup)**: Calories: 217; Fat: 4g; Protein: 7g; Carbohydrates: 39g; Fiber: 5g; Sodium: 88mg; Iron: 2mg

# Maple Oat Flax Granola

SERVES 6

**PREP TIME:** 5 minutes / **COOK TIME:** 30 to 45 minutes

Granola is typically high in refined sugar. This version has minimal added sugars (or none, if you swap out the maple syrup for dates).

2 tablespoons almond meal

2 tablespoons unsweetened finely shredded coconut

2 tablespoons flax meal

2 tablespoons avocado oil

2 tablespoons maple syrup, or 5 to 6 small dates, pitted

2 tablespoons brown rice flour

¼ teaspoon vanilla extract

Pinch sea salt

¾ cup rolled oats

1. Preheat the oven to 350°F.

2. In a food processor, combine the almond meal, coconut, flax meal, oil, and maple syrup and process until smooth.

3. Transfer the mixture to a bowl and stir in the flour, vanilla, and salt. Stir in the oats.

4. Spread the mixture evenly over a baking sheet and bake for 30 to 45 minutes, turning every 15 minutes, until golden brown. Let cool. Store in an airtight container.

**SUBSTITUTION TIP:** For variety, mix in ¼ cup raisins and ¼ cup sliced almonds when the granola is fresh out of the oven.

**Per Serving (about ¼ cup):** Calories: 150; Fat: 9g; Protein: 3g; Carbohydrates: 15g; Fiber: 2g; Sodium: 28mg; Iron: 1mg

# Blueberry Mango Smoothie

SERVES 2
**PREP TIME:** 5 minutes

Simple and quick, this refreshing smoothie is perfect for those mornings when you've just gotta get out the door. Frozen fruit comes in handy with this recipe! With 5 grams of fiber and plenty of protein, it's a sure way to keep you full until your next meal.

1½ cups unsweetened almond milk

1 small (6-inch) banana (best if frozen), chopped

1 cup loosely packed raw spinach

½ cup frozen wild blueberries

½ cup frozen mango chunks

2 small dates, pitted

1 tablespoon almond meal or almond butter

In a high-speed blender, combine the almond milk, banana, spinach, blueberries, mango, dates, and almond meal. Blend until smooth and creamy. Divide between two glasses and serve immediately.

**SUBSTITUTION TIP:** If you have fresh blueberries or mango, they're perfectly fine to use instead, as long as you have a frozen banana or a couple of ice cubes to make the smoothie thick, cool, and refreshing.

**Per Serving (1 cup):** Calories: 235; Fat: 12g; Protein: 6g; Carbohydrates: 35g; Fiber: 5g; Sodium: 73mg; Iron: 2mg

# Mock "Wheat Porridge"

SERVES 2

**PREP TIME:** 5 minutes / **COOK TIME:** 7 minutes

This grain-free hot cereal features cauliflower, a cruciferous vegetable that is naturally high in B vitamins and fiber. Its mild natural sweetness can make a comforting start to your day.

**2 cups chopped cauliflower**

**4 dates, pitted**

**¼ cup almond meal**

**2 teaspoons flax meal**

**½ cup unsweetened almond milk**

1. In a small pot with a steamer basket set inside, steam the cauliflower over boiling water, covered, for 7 minutes, or until soft.

2. Remove the steamer basket, transfer the cauliflower to a bowl, and mash it with a fork or whisk until the desired consistency is reached. Set aside.

3. In a high-speed blender, combine the dates, almond meal, and flax meal and blend until smooth. Add the mixture to the cauliflower and stir to combine.

4. Divide the porridge between two bowls and stir ¼ cup of the almond milk into each. Eat immediately or reheat when ready to serve.

**SUBSTITUTION TIP:** If you have a nut allergy, swap out the almond milk for unsweetened oat milk.

**Per Serving (1 cup)**: Calories: 188; Fat: 10g; Protein: 8g; Carbohydrates: 22g; Fiber: 8g; Sodium: 69mg; Iron: 2mg

# Tropical Overnight Oats

SERVES 1

**PREP TIME:** 2 minutes, plus overnight chilling

This tasty breakfast practically makes itself overnight. The oats soak up the milk, and the sweetness of the fruit blends for a delightful oat breakfast. Enjoy it served cold, straight out of the container, or warm it up if you desire.

½ cup frozen mango, cut into ½-inch cubes

½ medium banana, sliced

¼ cup rolled oats

1 tablespoon unsweetened finely shredded coconut

1 teaspoon chia seeds

⅛ teaspoon vanilla extract

Pinch sea salt

½ cup unsweetened almond milk

1. In a small glass jar with a lid, combine the mango, banana, oats, coconut, chia, vanilla, and salt and gently mix.

2. Add the almond milk and seal the jar.

3. Refrigerate overnight. Enjoy the following morning or store in the refrigerator for up to 4 days.

SUBSTITUTION TIP: If you are out of shredded coconut, you can swap in an equal amount of sliced almonds or almond meal.

Per Serving: Calories: 230; Fat: 14g; Protein: 6g; Carbohydrates: 33g; Fiber: 6g; Sodium: 185mg; Iron: 2mg

# Blueberry Flax Muffins

SERVES 12

**PREP TIME:** 10 minutes / **COOK TIME:** 20 to 25 minutes

These whole food muffins supply protein and fiber with no added sugars. Naturally sweetened fruit and accents of cinnamon, vanilla, and coconut make them a satisfying treat.

**12 small dates, pitted**

**½ cup flax meal**

**½ cup almond meal**

**¼ cup unsweetened shredded coconut**

**½ cup gluten-free flour**

**½ cup gluten-free rolled oats**

**1 tablespoon baking powder**

**¼ teaspoon sea salt**

**1⅓ cups unsweetened soy milk**

**¼ cup grape seed oil or avocado oil**

**1 medium egg**

**½ teaspoon vanilla extract**

**1 cup fresh blueberries**

1. Preheat the oven to 400°F. Line a 12-cup muffin tin with paper liners.

2. In a food processor, combine the dates, flax meal, almond meal, and coconut and process until well combined.

3. Transfer the mixture to a medium bowl. Stir the flour, oats, baking powder, and salt into the mixture.

4. In a separate bowl, combine the soy milk, oil, egg, and vanilla and stir until well blended.

5. Add the wet mixture to the dry mixture and stir until well combined. Let the mixture sit for 2 to 3 minutes, until it starts to thicken to a batter consistency.

6. Gently fold in the blueberries.

7. Scoop the batter evenly into the prepared muffin cups, using about ½ cup of the batter for each.

**8.** Bake for 20 to 25 minutes, until a toothpick inserted into the center of a muffin comes out clean.

**LOVING YOUR LEFTOVERS:** Enjoy a freshly baked muffin now, then freeze the rest for later. These are perfect for a grab-and-go breakfast. Simply thaw overnight in the fridge and reheat in the toaster oven or in the microwave for 30 seconds.

**Per Serving (1 muffin)**: Calories: 172; Fat: 10g; Protein: 5g; Carbohydrates: 17g; Fiber: 4g; Sodium: 189mg; Iron: 1mg

# Banana Berry Chia Pudding

**SERVES 2**

**PREP TIME:** 2 hours, plus overnight chilling

Chia is an amazing seed. When soaked, it can swell up to 10 times its original size. Just 1 tablespoon of chia contains more than 5 grams of fiber and 3 grams of protein (and it's a great plant source of omega-3s). This simple pudding is delicious, satisfying, and easy to make.

**1 cup unsweetened almond milk**

**4 tablespoons chia seeds**

**½ medium banana, sliced**

**2 tablespoons wild frozen blueberries**

**2 tablespoons sliced almonds**

**3 teaspoons raisins**

1. Divide the almond milk and chia seeds between two 8-ounce glass jars with tight-fitting lids or repurposed jam jars, seal tightly, and shake well.

2. Refrigerate for 2 hours, or until the mixture thickens.

3. Top each pudding with half the banana slices, 1 tablespoon of the blueberries, 1 tablespoon of the almonds, and 1½ teaspoons of the raisins.

4. Seal the jars tightly and store in the refrigerator overnight. Enjoy one the next morning. Store the remaining jar in the refrigerator for up to 4 days.

**SUBSTITUTION TIP:** If you have a nut allergy, swap the almonds for pumpkin seeds.

**Per Serving (1 cup)**: Calories: 273; Fat: 15g; Protein: 8g; Carbohydrates: 29g; Fiber: 10g; Sodium: 98mg; Iron: 4mg

# "Cocoa" Almond Smoothie

SERVES 2
**PREP TIME:** 2 minutes

Raspberries add a lovely zing to this carob and almond smoothie. Naturally sweet, low in fat, and high in fiber, carob is a great alternative to naturally caffeinated cocoa, which has been known to trigger GERD symptoms.

1¼ cups unsweetened almond milk

1 medium banana (frozen is best), sliced

½ cup raspberries

2 small dates, pitted

2 tablespoons unsweetened carob powder

2 tablespoons sliced almonds

1. In a high-speed blender, combine the almond milk, banana, raspberries, dates, carob, and almonds and blend until smooth and creamy.

2. Pour into two glasses and serve immediately.

**SUBSTITUTION TIP:** If you're really craving that chocolate flavor, swap out the carob for unsweetened cocoa powder.

**Per Serving (1 cup):** Calories: 208; Fat: 10g; Protein: 6g; Carbohydrates: 32g; Fiber: 8g; Sodium: 53mg; Iron: 1mg

# "Cheesy" Tofu Scramble with Spinach

SERVES 1

**PREP TIME:** 2 minutes / **COOK TIME:** 3 minutes

Tofu is an ideal plant-based substitute for eggs. It's a good source of protein, and when mashed with turmeric (a golden-hued spice), it can even replicate the look of scrambled eggs. To make this dish dairy-free, nutritional yeast is used as an alternative to Parmesan cheese.

**3 ounces firm tofu, mashed**

**⅛ teaspoon ground turmeric**

**1 tablespoon nutritional yeast**

**1 teaspoon almond meal**

**1½ teaspoons avocado oil, divided**

**Pinch sea salt**

**1 cup raw spinach**

1. In a bowl, mix the tofu with the turmeric so it resembles scrambled egg.

2. In a separate bowl, combine the nutritional yeast, almond meal, ½ teaspoon of oil, and the salt. Fold into the tofu mixture.

3. In a skillet, heat the remaining 1 teaspoon of oil over medium heat. Add the spinach and cook for about 2 minutes, stirring, until it turns bright green and wilts.

4. Add the tofu mixture and heat for another minute, until warmed through.

**PROTEIN SWAP:** If you are hankering for some real eggs, you can swap out the tofu for 1 whole egg and 3 egg whites. Keep the turmeric—it has anti-inflammatory properties!

**Per Serving**: Calories: 243; Fat: 16g; Protein: 19g; Carbohydrates: 9g; Fiber: 2g; Sodium: 191mg; Iron: 4mg

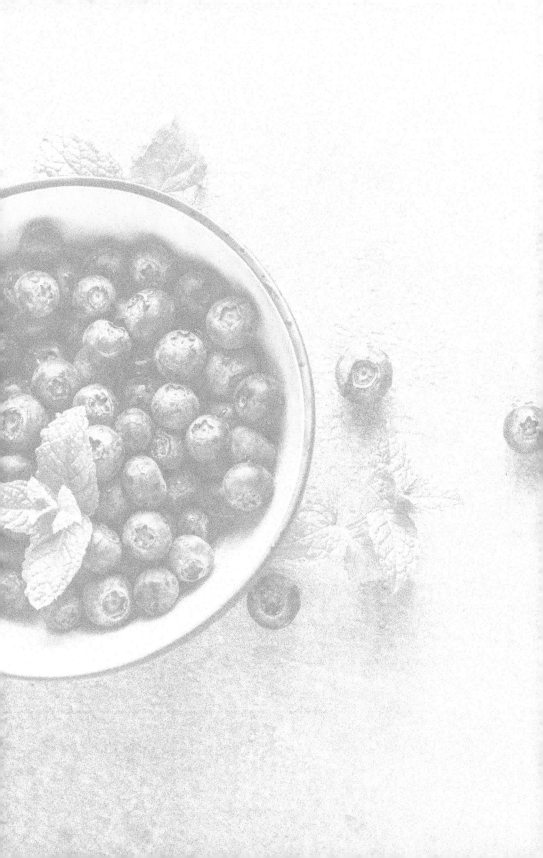

AVOCADO TOAST
WITH VEGAN
SPINACH-BASIL
PESTO
**PAGE 80**

# CHAPTER FIVE

# SIDES AND SNACKS

# Green Beans Almondine

**PREP TIME:** 1 minute / **COOK TIME:** 5 minutes

This side dish works with fresh, frozen, or leftover cooked green beans, and it complements a variety of main dishes. Low in calories and full of flavor, it's a quick and easy way to get your daily veggies.

2 teaspoons
avocado oil

2 teaspoons grated
fresh ginger, or
2 cubes frozen
ginger

¼ cup
sliced almonds

1 pound
steamed green
beans, chopped

1. In a skillet, heat the oil on medium heat. Add the ginger and cook for 2 to 3 minutes, stirring, until fragrant.

2. Add the almonds and toast in the pan for a couple of minutes, until just starting to turn golden.

3. Turn off the heat and mix in the green beans.

4. Serve warm or at room temperature.

**SUBSTITUTION TIP:** Swap out the ginger for garlic (if you don't suffer from GERD) for a different take on the dish.

**Per Serving**: Calories: 108; Fat: 6g; Protein: 5g; Carbohydrates: 10g; Fiber: 4g; Sodium: 7mg; Iron: 2mg

# Almond-Stuffed Dates with Coconut

SERVES 1

**PREP TIME:** 2 minutes

Naturally sweet dates are also a great source of fiber. An almond inside each of these simple-to-make snacks provides a delightfully crunchy surprise.

4 small dates, pitted

4 teaspoons unsweetened finely shredded coconut

4 whole raw almonds

1. With a small paring knife, slice each date open lengthwise.

2. Press 1 teaspoon of the coconut into the center of each date.

3. Place an almond into the center of the coconut.

4. Sprinkle any remaining coconut over the dates and enjoy.

**SUBSTITUTION TIP:** To add some variety, swap each almond for a cashew (or use 4 or 5 hulled pumpkin seeds per date).

**Per Serving**: Calories: 159; Fat: 7g; Protein: 2g; Carbohydrates: 25g; Fiber: 4g; Sodium: 2mg; Iron: 1mg

# Deviled Eggs

**PREP TIME:** 2 minutes

Deviled eggs may seem like a decadent treat, but you can enjoy them while eating alkaline. The homemade vegan mayonnaise in this recipe is simple to make. Using aquafaba, the liquid drained from a can of chickpeas, is a waste-reducing option. (Or use your favorite vegan mayo instead.)

**FOR THE DEVILED EGGS**

4 hard-boiled eggs

⅛ teaspoon sea salt

¼ teaspoon yellow mustard

**FOR THE CREAMY VEGAN MAYONNAISE**

¼ cup aquafaba (see Ingredient Tip, page 75)

⅛ teaspoon veggie seasoning salt, such as Mrs. Dash or Herbamare

1 cup avocado oil

To make the deviled eggs

1. Peel and slice each hard-boiled egg in half lengthwise. Scoop out the yolks and place the yolks in a small bowl. Set the egg whites aside. Mash the yolks with the salt and mustard and set aside.

To prepare the creamy vegan mayonnaise

2. In a food processor, combine the aquafaba and veggie seasoning salt and pulse for 30 seconds, until frothy.

3. With the food processor running on low, slowly drizzle in the oil and process until the liquid emulsifies into creamy mayonnaise.

4. Add 2 tablespoons of the mayonnaise to the egg yolks and mix well. (Transfer the remaining mayonnaise to a small jar with a tight-fitting lid and store in the refrigerator for 3 to 4 days.) Use a teaspoon to evenly scoop the egg yolk mixture into the cavity of each egg white and serve.

**SUBSTITUTION TIP:** If you don't want to use eggs, replace them with ¼ cup cooked shelled edamame and 4 button mushrooms, cleaned and stemmed. Mash the edamame with the sea salt and mustard and mix in the mayo, then scoop the mixture into the mushroom caps.

**INGREDIENT TIP:** Aquafaba is the viscous liquid in a can of chickpeas. In recipes, it can be used as a binder, similar to egg. That's what makes the vegan mayonnaise in these deviled eggs so thick and creamy. For this and other recipes calling for aquafaba, simply drain a can of chickpeas and reserve the liquid instead of discarding it. Store the liquid in an airtight container in the refrigerator for up to 3 days.

Per Serving (1 egg): Calories: 100; Fat: 8g; Protein: 6g; Carbohydrates: 1g; Fiber: 0g; Sodium: 149mg; Iron: 1mg

# Sweet Potato and Carrot Medallions

SERVES 6

**PREP TIME:** 5 minutes / **COOK TIME:** 35 to 45 minutes

A simple blend of sea salt, oil, and rosemary complements the naturally sweet flavors of sweet potatoes and carrots. These pigmented veggies provide immune-boosting vitamin C, as well as beta-carotene, an antioxidant that supports skin and eye health.

**2 large sweet potatoes, sliced into rounds**

**1 cup chopped carrots**

**4 teaspoons avocado oil or extra-virgin olive oil**

**2 teaspoons fresh rosemary**

**¼ teaspoon sea salt**

1. Preheat the oven to 400°F.

2. In a large bowl or resealable plastic bag, combine the sweet potatoes, carrots, oil, rosemary, and salt and mix until the carrots and sweet potatoes are well coated.

3. Pour the vegetables into a rectangular glass baking dish and arrange them in a single layer to cook evenly.

4. Roast for 35 to 45 minutes, until the thickest sweet potato rounds are soft; insert a paring knife to check.

**SUBSTITUTION TIP:** Try multicolored carrots (purple, white, and orange) to add color to your dish.

**Per Serving (½ cup)**: Calories: 95; Fat: 3g; Protein: 1g; Carbohydrates: 16g; Fiber: 3g; Sodium: 149mg; Iron: 1mg

# Carrot Fennel Slaw

SERVES 4

**PREP TIME:** 5 minutes

Prep this slaw in advance to allow the flavors to meld. Make it at the beginning of the week and store it in a sealed container in the refrigerator for a day or two before serving. It will be worth the wait.

**FOR THE SLAW**

1 cup chopped fennel

1 cup shredded carrots

¼ cup sliced almonds

3 tablespoons raisins

**FOR THE DIJON VINAIGRETTE**

1 tablespoon avocado oil

1 tablespoon freshly squeezed lemon juice

1 teaspoon apple cider vinegar

1 teaspoon Dijon or yellow mustard

1 teaspoon finely grated fresh ginger, or 1 cube frozen ginger

To make the slaw

1. In a medium bowl, toss the fennel, carrots, almonds, and raisins to combine; set aside.

To make the Dijon vinaigrette

2. In a small bowl, whisk together the oil, lemon juice, vinegar, mustard, and ginger until well combined.

3. Pour the dressing over the slaw and toss until evenly coated.

4. Serve cold or at room temperature. Store any leftovers in an airtight container in the refrigerator for up to 1 week.

**SUBSTITUTION TIP:** If you've already prepared a batch of Creamy Vegan Mayonnaise (see page 74), you can use the mayo in place of the vinaigrette and add lemon juice and mustard to taste.

**Per Serving (¾ cup):** Calories: 167; Fat: 9g; Protein: 5g; Carbohydrates: 19g; Fiber: 6g; Sodium: 195mg; Iron: 1mg

# Apple Slices with PB and Granola

SERVES 4

**PREP TIME:** 5 minutes

This straight-from-the-cupboard snack is a great way to enjoy your Maple Oat Flax Granola (page 60). It offers plenty of fiber and protein, too.

¼ **cup peanut butter**

**2 medium apples, cored and sliced**

½ **cup Maple Oat Flax Granola (page 60)**

1. Evenly spread a bit of peanut butter onto each apple slice.

2. Dip the peanut butter–coated side of each slice into the granola and serve.

**SUBSTITUTION TIP:** If you don't have granola on hand, you can make a muesli mixture to use in its place by combining 2 tablespoons gluten-free rolled oats, 1 tablespoon raisins, and 1 tablespoon sliced almonds.

**Per Serving (½ apple + 1 tablespoon peanut butter + 2 tablespoons granola):** Calories: 200; Fat: 12g; Protein: 5g; Carbohydrates: 19g; Fiber: 4g; Sodium: 195mg; Iron: 1mg

# Simple Hummus with Crudités

SERVES 1
**PREP TIME:** 5 minutes

Prepared with chickpeas, hummus is a great source of protein and fiber. Serve a couple of tablespoons of the hummus (store the rest) with your favorite combo of raw veggies, such as carrots, celery, and mushrooms.

**1 (15-ounce) can low-sodium chickpeas, drained and rinsed**

**3 tablespoons tahini**

**1 garlic clove, peeled**

**¼ cup freshly squeezed lemon juice**

**⅛ teaspoon sea salt**

**½ cup raw veggie slices or sticks**

1. In a high-speed blender, combine the chickpeas, tahini, garlic, lemon juice, and salt and blend until creamy.

2. Serve 2 tablespoons of the hummus with the veggies.

3. Store the remaining hummus in an airtight container in the refrigerator for up to 1 week.

**LOVING YOUR LEFTOVERS:** Use the remaining hummus as a dressing. Simply add the juice of 1 lime or lemon to ¼ cup of the hummus and mix in about 2 tablespoons warm water until thinned and well blended.

**Per Serving (2 tablespoons hummus + ½ cup vegetables)**: Calories: 152; Fat: 5g; Protein: 6g; Carbohydrates: 24g; Fiber: 7g; Sodium: 204mg; Iron: 1mg

# Avocado Toast with Vegan Spinach-Basil Pesto

**SERVES 2**

**PREP TIME:** 5 minutes

This simple variation on avocado toast is a great way to use leftover pesto from Vegan Spinach-Basil Pesto with Pasta (page 100). But if you haven't made that dish already, use the pesto recipe here.

**FOR THE AVOCADO TOAST**

½ medium avocado, halved

2 slices whole-grain bread, toasted

**FOR THE VEGAN SPINACH-BASIL PESTO**

4 cups baby spinach

1 cup fresh basil leaves

3 tablespoons extra-virgin olive oil

3 tablespoons walnuts

1 garlic clove, peeled, or 1 teaspoon garlic powder

⅛ teaspoon sea salt

To make the avocado toast

1. Cut slices into the flesh of the avocado and scoop out of the skin. Spread the avocado evenly over each piece of toast. Wrap the remaining avocado half (with pit intact) tightly in plastic wrap and refrigerate for up to 2 days.

To make the vegan spinach-basil pesto

2. In a high-speed blender, combine the spinach, basil, oil, walnuts, garlic, and salt and blend for 1 to 2 minutes, until the desired consistency is reached.

3. Top each avocado-smeared slice of toast with 1 tablespoon of the pesto and serve. Store the leftover pesto in an airtight container in the refrigerator for 4 to 5 days.

**SUBSTITUTION TIP:** Replace the pesto with a crunchy veggie such as sliced radishes or cucumber and top with cilantro.

**LOVING YOUR LEFTOVERS:** You can freeze a batch of pesto in an ice cube tray, then put the frozen pesto cubes in a tightly sealed freezer bag for up to 6 months. Simply reheat a cube whenever you need a convenient, portion-controlled flavor enhancer.

**Per Serving**: Calories: 205; Fat: 13g; Protein: 6g; Carbohydrates: 18g; Fiber: 6g; Sodium: 97mg; Iron: 2mg

# Cashew Almond Date Bars

SERVES 6
**PREP TIME:** 5 minutes

Yes, you can make your own energy bars. With whole food ingredients that contain plenty of fiber and protein, these healthy, convenient bars—with no added sugars or artificial ingredients—make the perfect snack.

**8 small dates, pitted**

**½ cup raw almonds**

**½ cup raw cashews**

**¼ cup flax meal**

**¼ cup unsweetened finely shredded coconut**

1. In a high-speed blender, combine the dates, almonds, cashews, flax meal, and coconut and blend until well combined.

2. Divide the mixture into 6 equal balls, each about 1½ inches in diameter. Mold each ball into a square or rectangle about ¼ inch thick.

3. Wrap each piece in plastic wrap and store in the refrigerator for up to 1 week or freeze for up to 3 months.

**MAKE IT EASIER:** Chop the dates by hand and mix all the ingredients together in a medium bowl for a simple trail mix instead. Divide evenly among 6 snack-size resealable plastic bags.

**Per Serving (1 bar)**: Calories: 176; Fat: 12g; Protein: 5g; Carbohydrates: 14g; Fiber: 4g; Sodium: 4mg; Iron: 1mg

# Hummus and Pesto Lettuce Wraps

**SERVES 1**

**PREP TIME:** 5 minutes

If you've prepared batches of hummus and pesto in the same week, use up any leftovers in this recipe. You'll make use of the lettuce in your crisper, too.

2 crisp romaine
lettuce leaves

2 tablespoons
Simple Hummus
(page 79)

2 tablespoons
Vegan Spinach-Basil
Pesto (page 100)

4 tablespoons
shredded carrots or
thinly sliced radishes

1. Place the lettuce leaves on a cutting board.

2. Spread 1 tablespoon of the hummus and 1 tablespoon of the pesto onto each lettuce leaf.

3. Top each with 2 tablespoons of the carrots.

4. Roll up and enjoy!

**SUBSTITUTION TIP:** Got one dip and not the other? Simply use one-quarter of a ripe avocado in its place.

**Per Serving**: Calories: 198; Fat: 12g; Protein: 7g; Carbohydrates: 20g; Fiber: 6g; Sodium: 168mg; Iron: 2mg

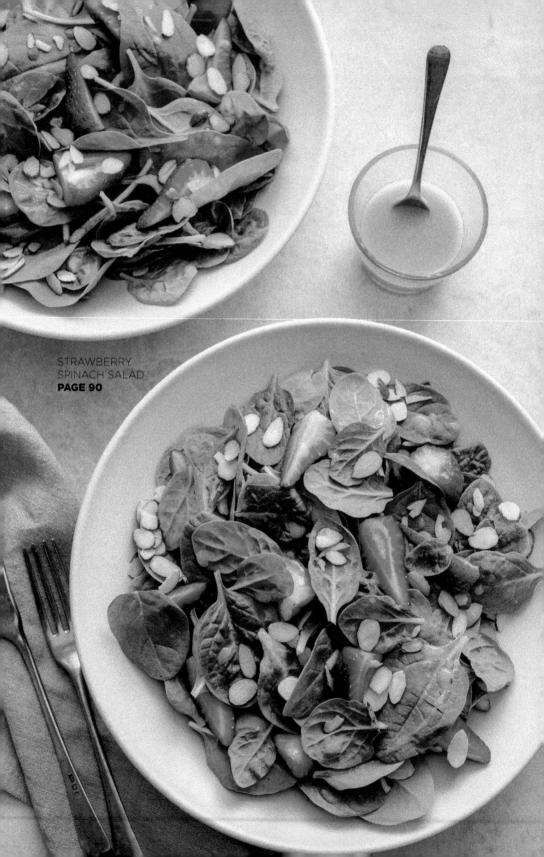

STRAWBERRY
SPINACH SALAD
**PAGE 90**

CHAPTER SIX

# SALADS AND SOUPS

# Curried Carrot and Raisin Tofu Salad

SERVES 6

**PREP TIME:** 10 minutes / **COOK TIME:** 3 minutes

Tofu contains all the essential amino acids and is a good source of non-dairy calcium. You can pan-fry or bake it, blend it into a smoothie, or use it as is. Because of its mild flavor and variety of available textures (silken, smooth, firm, or extra firm), it's a versatile ingredient for your cooking and meal-prep needs.

**8 ounces firm tofu, diced**

**½ cup shredded carrots**

**4 tablespoons chopped fresh basil, divided**

**2 tablespoons Creamy Vegan Mayonnaise (see page 74)**

**2 tablespoons raisins**

**2 tablespoons sliced almonds, divided**

**2 teaspoons curry powder or garam masala**

**½ teaspoon ground turmeric**

**⅛ teaspoon sea salt**

**8 ounces salad greens, for serving**

1. In a medium bowl, toss the tofu, carrots, 3 tablespoons of basil, the mayonnaise, raisins, 1 tablespoon of almonds, the curry powder, turmeric, and salt to combine.

2. In a nonstick pan, heat the mixture over low heat for 3 minutes or cover the bowl and microwave for 30 seconds.

3. Serve warm or at room temperature over a bed of greens. Garnish with the remaining 1 tablespoon each of almonds and basil.

**PROTEIN SWAP:** You can swap out the tofu for 8 ounces chopped cooked skinless chicken breast.

**Per Serving**: Calories: 144; Fat: 12g; Protein: 5g; Carbohydrates: 6g; Fiber: 2g; Sodium: 130mg; Iron: 1mg

# Mock Egg Salad

SERVES 4
**PREP TIME:** 5 minutes

Made with vegan mayonnaise and extra-firm tofu (I prefer the organic sprouted extra-firm tofu from Trader Joe's), this mock egg salad contains no animal-derived protein. The addition of anti-inflammatory turmeric produces a golden color to mimic that of an egg yolk.

**8 ounces extra-firm tofu**

**½ cup finely chopped celery**

**¼ teaspoon yellow mustard**

**¼ teaspoon ground turmeric**

**¼ teaspoon sea salt**

**2 tablespoons Creamy Vegan Mayonnaise (see page 74)**

**¼ cup finely chopped fresh basil**

**4 slices gluten-free bread, for serving (optional)**

**8 ounces leafy greens, for serving (optional)**

1. In a medium bowl, use a fork to mash the tofu so it resembles chopped hard-boiled egg.

2. Mix in the celery, mustard, turmeric, and salt.

3. Stir in the mayonnaise until well combined. Fold in the basil. Serve atop a slice of gluten-free bread or over a base of leafy greens and enjoy with a bowl of soup. Store leftovers in an airtight container in the refrigerator for 3 to 4 days.

**PROTEIN SWAP:** Want to use eggs instead? You can replace the tofu with 4 hard-boiled eggs, mashed.

**Per Serving**: Calories: 115; Fat: 9g; Protein: 8g; Carbohydrates: 1g; Fiber: 0g; Sodium: 175mg; Iron: 2mg

# Watermelon Tofu "Feta" Salad

SERVES 4

**PREP TIME:** 10 minutes

Watermelon is not only refreshing, it's also a good source of vitamin C. Paired with tofu "feta," it's a delicious choice. This vegan feta substitute is low in fat and provides 4 grams of protein per ounce, and the salad provides at least 100 milligrams of plant-based calcium per serving.

**FOR THE VEGAN TOFU "FETA"**

2 tablespoons freshly squeezed lemon juice

2 tablespoons avocado oil

1 teaspoon dried oregano

½ teaspoon dried thyme

¼ teaspoon garlic powder

¼ teaspoon sea salt

8 ounces firm tofu, cubed

**FOR THE SALAD**

¼ cup balsamic vinegar

8 dates, pitted

To make the vegan tofu "feta"

1. In a small bowl, combine the lemon juice, oil, oregano, thyme, garlic powder, and salt. Add the tofu and let it soak up the flavors while you make the salad.

To make the salad

2. In a high-speed blender, combine the vinegar and dates and blend until smooth.

3. Into each of four salad bowls, place 1 cup of the leafy greens. Add ¼ cup of the watermelon to each.

4. Using a slotted spoon, top each bowl with 2 tablespoons of the vegan feta. (Store the remaining vegan feta in an airtight container in the refrigerator for up to 5 days.)

4 cups crisp
leafy greens

1 cup cubed
watermelon

¼ cup chopped
fresh basil

5. Garnish evenly with the basil. Drizzle a tablespoon of the balsamic mixture onto each salad and serve.

**SUBSTITUTION TIP:** For a simpler option, you can swap out the Vegan Tofu "Feta" for an equal amount of cubed or crumbled tofu.

**Per Serving**: Calories: 147; Fat: 5g; Protein: 6g; Carbohydrates: 21g; Fiber: 3g; Sodium: 156mg; Iron: 7mg

# Strawberry Spinach Salad

**SERVES 4**

**PREP TIME:** 5 minutes

This salad's dark leafy greens pack plenty of iron, fiber, folate, and calcium. Strawberries add even more calcium, as well as vitamin C.

**FOR THE TURMERIC DIJON VINAIGRETTE**

3 tablespoons avocado oil

Juice of 1 small lemon

1 teaspoon Dijon or yellow mustard

¼ teaspoon ground turmeric

⅛ teaspoon sea salt

1 teaspoon maple syrup (optional)

**FOR THE SALAD**

4 cups baby spinach

1 cup halved strawberries

¼ cup sliced almonds

To make the turmeric Dijon vinaigrette

1. In a small bowl, whisk together the oil, lemon juice, mustard, turmeric, and salt until well combined. Add the maple syrup (if using) and mix well.

To make the salad

2. In a large bowl, toss the baby spinach, strawberries, and almonds.

3. Drizzle the dressing over the salad and gently toss to combine. Serve immediately. Or, if you are planning to serve later, store the undressed salad and the dressing in separate airtight containers in the refrigerator and add the dressing to the salad when ready to serve.

**VARIATION TIP:** Top each serving with 2 tablespoons Vegan Tofu "Feta" (see page 88) to get an additional 4 grams of protein.

Per Serving: Calories: 160; Fat: 14g; Protein: 3g; Carbohydrates: 6g; Fiber: 3g; Sodium: 30mg; Iron: 2mg

# Creamy Zucchini Soup

**PREP TIME:** 5 minutes / **COOK TIME:** 25 minutes

This low-calorie, nutrient-dense soup is loaded with vegetables and flavor. Nearly 6 grams of fiber and 6 grams of protein mean it's satisfying, too. Adding cooked quinoa lends the soup even more texture and protein.

**2 tablespoons avocado oil**

**¼ teaspoon dried oregano**

**¼ teaspoon dried thyme**

**⅛ teaspoon sea salt**

**1 large onion, chopped**

**2 large zucchini, peeled and chopped**

**1 cup low-sodium vegetable broth**

**1 cup water**

**1 cup baby spinach**

**6 large fresh basil leaves**

**⅓ cup cooked quinoa (optional)**

**Juice of 1 lemon**

1. In a soup pot, heat the oil on medium heat for 1 minute, then add the oregano, thyme, and salt and cook for 30 seconds.

2. Add the onion, cover, and cook for 7 to 8 minutes, stirring regularly, until softened.

3. Add the zucchini. Cook for another 12 minutes, or until the zucchini is soft.

4. Add the broth and water and cook for another 3 minutes, until warmed.

5. Toss in the spinach and basil and cook until just wilted.

6. Transfer the mixture to a food processor and process until pureed.

7. Add the quinoa (if using). Season with the lemon juice and serve.

**SUBSTITUTION TIP:** If you suffer from GERD, replace the onions with an equal amount of chopped fennel. The fennel becomes soft and translucent just like the onion. It's a different flavor, but adds a similar textural appeal.

**Per Serving**: Calories: 140; Fat: 11g; Protein: 3g; Carbohydrates: 10g; Fiber: 3g; Sodium: 201mg; Iron: 1mg

# Sweet Pumpkin and Apple Soup

SERVES 2

**PREP TIME:** 5 minutes / **COOK TIME:** 25 minutes

This soup's got the benefit of vitamins A, C, and E—all great for immunity—plus beta-carotene for skin and eye health. It's also packed with fiber.

1 medium apple, cored and sliced

½ cup chopped fennel

1½ cups water, divided

1 cup canned unsweetened pumpkin puree

¾ cup low-sodium vegetable broth

4 small dates, pitted

2 teaspoons grated fresh ginger, or 2 cubes frozen ginger

¼ teaspoon ground cinnamon

¼ teaspoon curry powder

⅛ teaspoon dried thyme

⅛ teaspoon sea salt

⅛ teaspoon ground cumin

1. In a saucepan, combine the apples, fennel, and ½ cup of water. Cover and cook on low for about 25 minutes, until the apples and fennel are softened.

2. In a food processor, combine the apple-fennel mixture, pumpkin, remaining 1 cup of water, the broth, dates, ginger, cinnamon, curry powder, thyme, salt, and cumin. Process until pureed.

3. Pour the soup into two bowls and garnish each with 2 teaspoons of the raisins and 1 teaspoon of the toasted fennel seeds.

4. Serve immediately or let cool and serve at room temperature.

**4 teaspoons raisins, for garnish**

**2 teaspoons fennel seeds, toasted, for garnish**

**INGREDIENT SWAP:** You can replace the pumpkin puree with 1 medium sweet potato, baked and peeled.

**Per Serving**: Calories: 221; Fat: 5g; Protein: 6g; Carbohydrates: 46g; Fiber: 11g; Sodium: 260mg; Iron: 4mg

# Roasted Carrot-Tomato Soup

**SERVES 2**

**PREP TIME:** 5 minutes / **COOK TIME:** 35 minutes

Tomatoes provide fiber, potassium, and vitamin C. Carrots are rich in beta-carotene. Together they provide a nourishing base for this zesty soup. Made with ingredients straight from the cupboard, it's a convenient, cost-effective option.

1 (15-ounce) can no-sodium-added diced tomatoes, drained

¾ cup chopped carrots

1 tablespoon avocado oil

¼ teaspoon sea salt

1 cup water

½ cup low-sodium vegetable broth

2 tablespoons chopped fresh cilantro

1 tablespoon freshly squeezed lemon juice

1. Preheat the oven to 400°F.

2. In a glass baking dish, combine the tomatoes, carrots, oil, and salt and mix well.

3. Bake the tomato-carrot mixture for 35 minutes, or until caramelized, then carefully transfer to a food processor.

4. Add the water and broth, and puree until smooth.

5. Garnish with the cilantro and add the lemon juice to taste.

**LOVING YOUR LEFTOVERS:** The baked tomato-carrot mixture makes a nice salsa-like garnish for baked fish or bean tacos, or is great served over wild rice or quinoa. Make a double batch, use half for the soup, and store the other half to use in other dishes throughout the week.

**Per Serving**: Calories: 131; Fat: 7g; Protein: 2g; Carbohydrates: 15g; Fiber: 4g; Sodium: 259mg; Iron: 2mg

# Zucchini, Bell Pepper, and Basil Soup

SERVES 2

**PREP TIME:** 5 minutes

Cold soups can be convenient, refreshing, and nourishing. They are also a great way to use a variety of veggies, and they offer a savory alternative to a green smoothie. This soup contains vitamin C, potassium, and digestion-friendly basil. With 8 grams of protein and 10 grams of fiber, it's sure to satisfy.

2 large
zucchini, chopped

1 medium avocado

1 medium
bell pepper

½ cup low-sodium
vegetable broth

½ cup water

¼ cup
chopped fennel

6 fresh basil leaves,
plus 2 small leaves
for garnish

2 teaspoons
chopped
fresh rosemary

1 garlic clove,
peeled, or 1 cube
frozen garlic

⅛ teaspoon sea salt

1½ teaspoons hulled
pumpkin seeds,
toasted, for garnish

1. In a high-speed blender or food processor, combine the zucchini, avocado, bell pepper, broth, water, fennel, basil, rosemary, garlic, and salt and blend until pureed.

2. Pour the soup into bowls. Garnish each with a small basil leaf and the pumpkin seeds, and serve.

**SUBSTITUTION TIP:** You can swap out the basil for 2 tablespoons fresh cilantro and use 2 small sprigs for the garnish. It adds an equally refreshing appeal.

**Per Serving**: Calories: 224; Fat: 14g; Protein: 8g; Carbohydrates: 24g; Fiber: 10g; Sodium: 240mg; Iron: 3mg

# Spring Greens with Radish, Zucchini, and Dijon Vinaigrette

**SERVES 4**

**PREP TIME:** 5 minutes

This classic side salad will enliven any meal. For variety, try different greens like romaine or arugula, and swap the radish and zucchini for any crunchy vegetables you have on hand. Dijon dressing adds tang.

**4 cups loosely packed spring greens**

**½ cup sliced radishes**

**½ cup sliced zucchini**

**¼ cup Turmeric Dijon Vinaigrette (see page 90)**

1. In a large bowl, toss the greens with the radishes and zucchini.

2. Drizzle with the vinaigrette and toss to coat well.

**LOVING YOUR LEFTOVERS:** If you are eating for one, add approximately 2 teaspoons dressing per 1 cup prepared salad. Refrigerate the remaining salad and dressing separately in sealed containers.

Per Serving: Calories: 108; Fat: 10g; Protein: 2g; Carbohydrates: 4.3g; Fiber: 2g; Sodium: 146mg; Iron: 2mg

# Chickpea Rainbow Salad

**SERVES 4**

**PREP TIME:** 5 minutes

Tangy and refreshing, the mango-citrus salsa in this recipe is best when it's allowed to marinate for several hours or up to overnight. When the salsa is ready, mix it with the chickpeas and bell peppers for a heart-healthy combo that's bursting with flavor.

**FOR THE MANGO-CITRUS SALSA**

2 cups chopped mango

1 cup chopped fennel

⅓ cup chopped scallions

¼ cup fresh chopped basil

3 tablespoons freshly squeezed lemon juice

¼ teaspoon sea salt

**FOR THE RAINBOW SALAD**

1 (15-ounce) can low-sodium chickpeas, drained (liquid reserved) and rinsed

½ cup chopped bell pepper

1 teaspoon chopped fresh cilantro, for garnish

**To make the mango-citrus salsa**

1. In a medium bowl, combine the mango, fennel, scallions, basil, lemon juice, and salt and toss well. For best results, cover and refrigerate for several hours or up to overnight to let the flavors meld.

**To make the rainbow salad**

2. In a large bowl, combine the chickpeas, bell pepper, and ¼ cup of the salsa. (Store the remaining salsa in an airtight container in the refrigerator for 5 to 7 days.)

3. Garnish the salad with the cilantro and serve.

**LOVING YOUR LEFTOVERS:** Save the liquid from the canned chickpeas (known as aquafaba) in an airtight container in the refrigerator for up to 2 days so you can use it to make Creamy Vegan Mayonnaise (see page 74).

**Per Serving**: Calories: 126; Fat: 2g; Protein: 6g; Carbohydrates: 24g; Fiber: 6g; Sodium: 366mg; Iron: 1mg

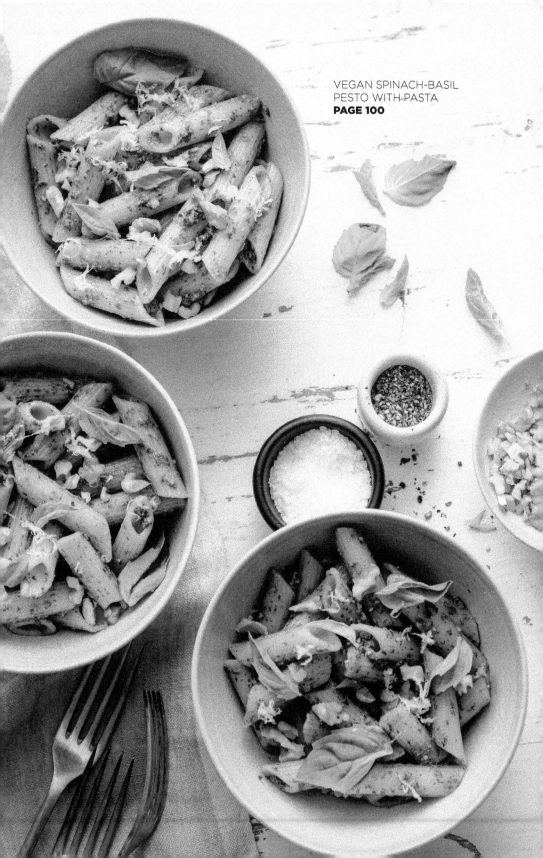

VEGAN SPINACH-BASIL
PESTO WITH PASTA
**PAGE 100**

# MAINS

# Vegan Spinach-Basil Pesto with Pasta

SERVES 4

**PREP TIME:** 10 minutes / **COOK TIME:** 10 minutes

The hearty pesto in this dish contains less salt and oil than most processed versions. Baby spinach provides an extra health boost.

**2 cups dried gluten-free pasta**

**3 cups packed baby spinach**

**½ cup packed fresh basil**

**3 tablespoons avocado oil**

**3 tablespoons walnut pieces**

**1 to 2 garlic cloves, peeled**

**⅛ teaspoon sea salt**

1. Bring a pot of water to a boil and cook the pasta according to the package instructions. Drain, transfer to a large bowl, and set aside.

2. In a food processor, combine the spinach, basil, oil, walnuts, garlic, and salt and pulse for 20 to 30 seconds, until the desired consistency is reached. Toss the pesto with the cooked pasta and serve.

**VARIATION TIP:** If you are seeking something tangier (and don't suffer from GERD), you can add 1 tablespoon freshly squeezed Meyer lemon juice. You can also replace the walnuts with ¼ cup sliced almonds.

**SUBSTITUTION TIP:** Omit the pasta and scoop 1 rounded tablespoon of the pesto into cremini mushroom caps (rinsed and dried) for a fun, tasty appetizer or snack.

**Per Serving**: Calories: 320; Fat: 15g; Protein: 6g; Carbohydrates: 43g; Fiber: 7g; Sodium: 24mg; Iron: 2mg

# Seasoned Lentils over Rice

**SERVES 4**
**PREP TIME:** 5 minutes / **COOK TIME:** 15 minutes

Lentils are classified as both a carbohydrate and a protein. As a complex carb, this legume contains heart-healthy B vitamins and a good amount of fiber. This dish provides plenty of protein and complex carbs.

**FOR THE TACO SPICE BLEND**

4 teaspoons garlic powder

2 teaspoons ground cumin

2 teaspoons dried oregano

2 teaspoons ground cinnamon

1 teaspoon sea salt

**FOR THE LENTILS AND RICE**

2 cups cooked lentils

2 teaspoons olive oil or avocado oil

2 cups cooked brown rice

To make the taco spice blend

1. In a small bowl, mix the garlic powder, cumin, oregano, cinnamon, and salt.

To make the lentils and rice

2. In a large bowl, toss the lentils, oil, and 1 tablespoon of the taco spice blend. (Store the remaining taco spice blend in a small jar in the cupboard for another use.)

3. Serve ½ cup of the seasoned lentils over ½ cup of the rice.

**VARIATION TIP:** Add 1 cup steamed veggies (your choice) to make this a complete meal.

**Per Serving**: Calories: 264; Fat: 4g; Protein: 12g; Carbohydrates: 47g; Fiber: 8g; Sodium: 153mg; Iron: 4mg

# Black Bean Veggie Tostada

**SERVES 4**

**PREP TIME:** 5 minutes / **COOK TIME:** 20 minutes

Black beans can be used in soups, casseroles, tacos—you name it. And like lentils, they are a fiber-rich protein. With B vitamins, potassium, and iron, canned black beans are a convenient source of essential nutrients. Bonus: This dish has 14 grams of protein and a whopping 5 grams of iron per serving.

1½ tablespoons avocado oil or extra-virgin olive oil

½ large onion, sliced

¼ teaspoon dried thyme

¼ teaspoon dried oregano

1 large zucchini, sliced

1 cup sliced mushrooms

¼ cup canned low-sodium diced tomatoes

1 (15-ounce) can low-sodium black beans, drained (liquid reserved) and rinsed

1 tablespoon Taco Spice Blend (see page 101)

4 (6-inch) corn tortillas

1 avocado, sliced

1. In a skillet, heat the oil on medium for 1 minute. Add the onion, thyme, and oregano and cook for 5 to 7 minutes, until softened.

2. Mix in the zucchini, mushrooms, and tomatoes and cook for another 5 to 7 minutes, until softened.

3. Add the beans, ¼ cup of the reserved liquid from the can, and the taco spice blend and heat until warmed.

4. Warm the corn tortillas in a toaster oven or on the stove until lightly browned.

5. With a slotted spoon, scoop the black beans into the heated tortillas, dividing them evenly.

6. Garnish with the avocado slices and serve.

**SUBSTITUTION TIP:** You can swap out the black beans for cooked lentils if you prefer a legume.

**Per Serving (1 tostada):** Calories: 322; Fat: 12g; Protein: 14g; Carbohydrates: 43g; Fiber: 12g; Sodium: 294mg; Iron: 5mg

# Quinoa Black Bean Veggie Bowl

**SERVES 4**

**PREP TIME:** 2 minutes / **COOK TIME:** 20 minutes

Quinoa contains all nine essential amino acids.

1 cup canned black
beans, drained
and rinsed

1 to 2 teaspoons
Taco Spice Blend
(see page 101)

4 cups chopped
Tuscan kale

Sea salt

1 cup sliced
mushrooms

1 cup cooked quinoa

½ cup shredded
carrots

1 medium
avocado, sliced

¼ cup Simple
Hummus (page 79)

Juice of
½ medium lime

1 to 3 tablespoons
warm water

3 tablespoons
shelled pistachios

8 teaspoons pico
de gallo

4 teaspoons
chopped
fresh cilantro

1. In a small bowl, mix the black beans and taco spice blend.

2. Put the kale in a large bowl and lightly season with salt. Using your hands, massage the kale until softened slightly. Divide the kale, mushrooms, bean mixture, quinoa, carrots, and avocado evenly among four bowls.

3. In a small bowl, mix the hummus with the lime juice, and add the warm water, 1 tablespoon at a time, until it has thinned to a dressing consistency. Drizzle 1 tablespoon of the dressing onto each veggie bowl.

4. Garnish each bowl evenly with the pistachios, pico de gallo, and cilantro.

**LOVING YOUR LEFTOVERS:** If you know you won't be serving all four bowls, store the undressed ingredients and the dressing in separate airtight containers in the refrigerator for up to 4 days.

**Per Serving**: Calories: 290; Fat: 12g; Protein: 12g; Carbohydrates: 47g; Fiber: 12g; Sodium: 508mg; Iron: 4mg

# Zucchini Frittata with Tofu "Ricotta" and Lemon

**PREP TIME:** 2 minutes / **COOK TIME:** 20 minutes

This frittata uses vegan tofu "ricotta" as an alternative to cheese. With the benefit of protein and plant-based calcium, tofu-based "cheese" is a healthy alternative to traditional creamy cheeses.

**FOR THE VEGAN TOFU "RICOTTA"**

8 ounces firm tofu, crumbled

2 tablespoons avocado oil

1 tablespoon freshly squeezed lemon juice

⅛ teaspoon sea salt

⅛ teaspoon ground nutmeg

**FOR THE FRITTATA**

Nonstick cooking spray

3 medium eggs, beaten

2 tablespoons freshly squeezed lemon juice

¼ teaspoon ground nutmeg

To make the vegan tofu "ricotta"

1. In a medium bowl, combine the tofu, oil, lemon juice, salt, and nutmeg. Mix well and set aside.

To make the frittata

2. Preheat the oven to 350°F. Spray an 8- or 9-inch square glass baking dish with cooking spray.

3. In a bowl, combine the tofu "ricotta," eggs, lemon juice, and nutmeg and mix well. Transfer to the prepared baking dish.

4. Top with the zucchini slices and drizzle with the oil.

5. Bake for 20 to 25 minutes, until the eggy batter is firm.

1 cup sliced zucchini

2 teaspoons avocado oil

1 teaspoon Taco Spice Blend (see page 101)

2 tablespoons chopped scallion

6. Garnish with the taco spice blend and scallions.

**VARIATION TIP:** To keep this fritatta on the mild side, replace the Taco Spice Blend with additional nutmeg to taste and swap out the scallions for chopped basil.

..................................................................

**Per Serving**: Calories: 224; Fat: 17g; Protein: 13g; Carbohydrates: 4g; Fiber: 1g; Sodium: 182mg; Iron: 2mg

# Seasoned Lentil Tacos with Bell Peppers and Onions

SERVES 4

**PREP TIME:** 2 minutes / **COOK TIME:** 20 minutes

Compared with an orange, bell peppers contain three times more vitamin C, which aids in iron absorption. This dish contains 5 milligrams of iron (25 percent of your recommended daily intake). Even better news, you get to enjoy two tacos, which together have fewer than 300 calories!

**2 cups cooked lentils**

**1 teaspoon Taco Spice Blend (see page 101)**

**2 teaspoons extra-virgin olive oil**

**1 medium onion, sliced**

**2 cups sliced bell peppers (frozen is fine)**

**8 (6-inch) corn tortillas**

**2 tablespoons chopped fresh cilantro**

1. In a small bowl, mix the lentils and taco spice blend.

2. In a skillet, heat the oil on low. Add the onion and bell peppers and cook for about 15 minutes, until the bell peppers are soft and the onion is translucent.

3. Add the seasoned lentils and cook for another 3 minutes, until warmed through.

4. Evenly divide the lentil-vegetable mixture among the tortillas. Garnish with the cilantro and serve.

**SUBSTITUTION TIP:** To keep it on the mild side, replace the Taco Spice Blend with nutmeg to taste and swap out the onion for chopped fresh basil.

**Per Serving (2 tacos)**: Calories: 267; Fat: 4g; Protein: 13g; Carbohydrates: 48g; Fiber: 10g; Sodium: 174mg; Iron: 5mg

# Vegan Pumpkin Chili

SERVES 4

**PREP TIME:** 10 minutes / **COOK TIME:** 20 minutes

This chili, packed with pumpkin, beans, and bell peppers, contains plenty of plant-based goodness, including fiber, B vitamins, potassium, and antioxidants such as beta-carotene. Each serving meets 18 percent of your recommended daily iron.

1 tablespoon avocado oil

1 cup diced celery

⅛ teaspoon sea salt

1 (15-ounce) can low-sodium black beans, drained and rinsed

1 cup canned pumpkin puree

1 cup yellow corn kernels

½ cup low-sodium vegetable broth

½ cup water

2 teaspoons grated fresh ginger, or 2 cubes frozen ginger

¼ teaspoon ground cinnamon

¼ teaspoon dried thyme

½ teaspoon ground cumin

Juice of ½ lemon

1. In a pan, heat the oil over medium heat for 1 minute. Add the celery and salt and cook for 5 minutes, or until the celery is soft.

2. Add the black beans, pumpkin, corn, broth, water, ginger, cinnamon, thyme, and cumin and heat until thoroughly warmed.

3. Squeeze in the lemon juice and serve.

**INGREDIENT TIP:** Frozen cubes of crushed ginger are available in certain supermarkets and online, and make a convenient way to add fresh ginger without the hassle of peeling and grating it. Each cube is approximately 1 teaspoon for ease of measurement. Dorot Gardens is one brand of these easy-to-use cubes.

**Per Serving**: Calories: 202; Fat: 4g; Protein: 8g; Carbohydrates: 35g; Fiber: 12g; Sodium: 393mg; Iron: 3mg

# Sautéed Eggplant with Quinoa and Mango-Citrus Salsa

SERVES 4

**PREP TIME:** 10 minutes / **COOK TIME:** 25 minutes

Quinoa adds a slightly nutty flavor and crunch to complement the savory eggplant in this dish, and the Mango-Citrus Salsa adds a refreshing tang. This hearty combo provides magnesium and potassium (both nutrients that aid in blood pressure control) and immune-boosting vitamin C.

2 teaspoons
extra-virgin olive oil

1 tablespoon Taco
Spice Blend (see
page 101)

1 medium
eggplant, chopped

4 cups raw spinach

2 cups
cooked quinoa

1 cup Mango-Citrus
Salsa (see page 97)

1. In a skillet, heat the oil and the taco spice blend over medium heat. Add the eggplant and cook, turning the pieces occasinally, for about 25 minutes, until thoroughly softened.

2. Add the spinach to the pan with the eggplant and cook until the spinach wilts.

3. Divide the quinoa among four bowls and spoon the eggplant mixture over the quinoa.

4. Garnish with the salsa.

**VARIATION TIP:** Mix a pinch of sea salt into the prepared quinoa. It will remove any bitterness and enliven the sweet, nutty flavor of the grain.

**Per Serving**: Calories: 240; Fat: 5g; Protein: 8g; Carbohydrates: 45g; Fiber: 11g; Sodium: 277mg; Iron: 3mg

# Vegan Stuffed Eggplant

**SERVES 4**

**PREP TIME:** 10 minutes / **COOK TIME:** 30 minutes

This dish is hearty yet surprisingly low in calories.

**1 large eggplant, cut in half lengthwise**

**3 tablespoons extra-virgin olive oil or avocado oil, divided**

**⅛ teaspoon sea salt**

**2 garlic cloves, crushed, or 2 frozen garlic cubes**

**1 teaspoon Taco Spice Blend (see page 101)**

**2 cups sliced mushrooms**

**1 cup canned low-sodium diced tomatoes**

**1 cup canned low-sodium chickpeas, drained and rinsed**

1. Preheat the oven to 425°F. Line a baking sheet with aluminum foil.

2. Place the eggplant on the baking sheet and brush each side with 1½ teaspoons of oil. Sprinkle both sides with the salt.

3. Place the eggplant halves cut-side down on the baking sheet and bake for 30 to 40 minutes, until the flesh softens and the outer skin puckers.

4. Meanwhile, in a skillet, heat the remaining 1 tablespoon of oil on medium heat. Add the garlic and taco spice blend and cook for 2 minutes.

5. Add the mushrooms and tomatoes to the skillet and cook for another 10 minutes, or until the mushrooms are soft.

6. Add the chickpeas and cook for another 3 minutes, or until warmed through. Remove from the heat and cover.

7. Divide the mushroom mixture between the eggplant halves and cut each in half to make four servings.

Per Serving: Calories: 183; Fat: 8g; Protein: 6g; Carbohydrates: 23g; Fiber: 9g; Sodium: 365mg; Iron: 2mg

# Fennel-Seasoned Falafel with Hummus Dressing

SERVES 4

**PREP TIME:** 10 minutes / **COOK TIME:** 20 minutes

Baked, not fried, this heart-healthy falafel provides 9 grams of fiber and 13 grams of protein in each serving.

1½ cups arugula

1 cup canned low-sodium chickpeas, drained (liquid reserved) and rinsed

¾ cup almond meal

¼ cup chopped fennel

2 tablespoons tahini

Juice of 1 lemon, divided

1 teaspoon low-sodium soy sauce or Bragg Liquid Aminos

½ cup Simple Hummus (page 79) or store-bought hummus

1. Preheat the oven to 350°F. Line a baking sheet with parchment paper or aluminum foil, or grease it with oil.

2. In a food processor, combine the arugula, chickpeas, almond meal, fennel, tahini, half the lemon juice, and the soy sauce.

3. Roll the mixture into 1½-inch balls (I use a 1-ounce mini scoop) and place them 2 inches apart on the prepared baking sheet. Bake for 20 minutes, or until golden.

4. In a small bowl, mix the hummus and remaining lemon juice. Add water, 1 tablespoon at a time, until the desired consistency is reached.

5. Drizzle 1 to 2 teaspoons of the hummus mixture over the falafel and serve.

**VARIATION TIP:** Use nonstick cooking spray to lightly coat the falafel balls before baking to increase their golden crispness.

**Per Serving**: Calories: 307; Fat: 19g; Protein: 13g; Carbohydrates: 27g; Fiber: 9g; Sodium: 362mg; Iron: 3mg

# Zucchini and Pesto Grain Bowl

SERVES 4
**PREP TIME:** 5 minutes

Whether you slice it or spiralize it, zucchini has the benefit of bone-protective nutrients including calcium, magnesium, and potassium.

4 cups arugula

4 cups zucchini noodles (spiralized or thinly sliced)

2 cups cooked quinoa

½ cup Vegan Spinach-Basil Pesto (see page 100)

½ cup sliced cherry tomatoes or drained canned low-sodium diced tomatoes

4 tablespoons hulled pumpkin seeds

1. Divide the arugula evenly among four bowls.

2. In each bowl, layer 1 cup of the zucchini noodles, ½ cup of the quinoa, 2 tablespoons of the pesto, and 2 tablespoons of the tomatoes.

3. Garnish each with 1 tablespoon of the pumpkin seeds.

**SUBSTITUTION TIP:** If you have a tomato allergy or GERD, replace the tomatoes with an equal amount of reheated cooked carrots.

**Per Serving**: Calories: 245; Fat: 13g; Protein: 9g; Carbohydrates: 24g; Fiber: 5g; Sodium: 34mg; Iron: 3mg

# Vegan Cauliflower-and-Mushroom Lasagna

SERVES 6

**PREP TIME:** 10 minutes / **COOK TIME:** 30 minutes

No cheese, no problem! That's because this vegan lasagna uses vegan "ricotta" made from tofu to give it a dairy-free ricotta appeal. Seasoned tomatoes, mushrooms, and spinach add veggie-based goodness.

1 large head cauliflower, sliced into ¼-inch-thick disks

1 tablespoon avocado oil

⅛ teaspoon sea salt

1 (15-ounce) can low-sodium diced tomatoes, with their juices

1 teaspoon Taco Spice Blend (see page 101)

1 recipe Vegan Tofu "Ricotta" (see page 104)

4 cooked lasagna noodles

2 cups chopped spinach

1 cup sliced mushrooms

1½ tablespoons vegan Parmesan (page 68, step 2)

1. Preheat the oven to 425°F.

2. Place the cauliflower in a layer over the bottom of a baking pan, brush evenly with the oil, sprinkle with the salt, and bake for 30 minutes, or until softened but still slightly firm (al dente).

3. While the cauliflower is baking, in a bowl, mix the tomatoes and their juices and the taco spice blend.

4. Remove the cauliflower from the oven and layer the vegan "ricotta," lasagna noodles, spinach, mushrooms, and seasoned tomatoes on top.

5. Bake for another 20 minutes, then garnish with the Parmesan and serve.

**SUBSTITUTION TIP:** For a less-refined option, replace the lasagna noodles with 2 cups cooked quinoa.

**Per Serving**: Calories: 228; Fat: 11g; Protein: 11g; Carbohydrates: 23g; Fiber: 5g; Sodium: 417mg; Iron: 3mg

# Almond-Crusted Tofu with Mango-Citrus Salsa

SERVES 4
**PREP TIME:** 5 to 7 minutes / **COOK TIME:** 20 minutes

This tasty dish provides a nice balance of fruit, veggies, protein, and starch, with some healthy fats to boot. With 26 grams of protein and 4 grams of fiber, it is sure to satisfy!

¼ cup rice flour

2 medium eggs, well beaten

½ cup sliced almonds, crushed

15 ounces firm tofu, sliced

1 tablespoon extra-virgin olive oil

2 cups steamed broccoli

½ cup Mango-Citrus Salsa (see page 97)

1. Place the rice flour, eggs, and almonds in three separate small bowls.

2. Dip each slice of tofu into the rice flour, then in the egg, and finally coat with the crushed almonds. Set on a plate and repeat to coat the remaining tofu.

3. In a skillet, heat the oil over medium-high heat for 30 to 45 seconds.

4. Pan-fry the tofu slices in the hot oil for 4 to 5 minutes on each side, until golden.

5. Serve the tofu with the steamed broccoli and mango-citrus salsa.

**PROTEIN SWAP:** Swap out the tofu for 2 salmon fillets (approximately 1 pound total) and coat them as above. Instead of pan-frying the salmon, bake at 400°F for approximately 12 minutes, until the flesh is soft and flakes easily with a fork. Divide each fillet into two equal pieces and serve. (It is easier to divide the fish into equal portions after it's cooked.)

**Per Serving**: Calories: 372; Fat: 23g; Protein: 26g; Carbohydrates: 18g; Fiber: 4g; Sodium: 66mg; Iron: 5mg

BLUEBERRY-BANANA
SOFT SERVE
**PAGE 116**

# CHAPTER EIGHT

# DESSERTS

# Blueberry-Banana Soft Serve

SERVES 2

**PREP TIME:** 5 minutes

This soft serve is a super easy alternative to ice cream. With only three ingredients, it's a snap to make (and it doesn't require any freezing time). Enjoy it right away for a refreshing snack or dessert.

1 small ripe banana

1 cup frozen wild blueberries

1 teaspoon freshly squeezed lemon juice

In a high-speed blender or food processor, combine banana, blueberries, and lemon juice. Blend until creamy and smooth. Enjoy immediately.

**LOVING YOUR LEFTOVERS:** You can enjoy one serving now and freeze the rest. Use it as a base for a smoothie by adding 1 cup unsweetened almond milk and ½ cup fresh or frozen fruit.

**Per Serving (½ cup)**: Calories: 81; Fat: 1g; Protein: 1g; Carbohydrates: 20g; Fiber: 3g; Sodium: 3mg; Iron: 1mg

# Baked Apple Crumble

SERVES 4

**PREP TIME:** 5 minutes / **COOK TIME:** 20 to 25 minutes

If you love apple pie, you'll love this simple (gluten-free!) dessert. You get a whole serving of fresh fruit and minimal fat and sugar. Be sure to use foil to keep the fruit moist as it bakes.

**4 small apples**

**¼ cup gluten-free rolled oats**

**¼ cup unsweetened shredded coconut**

**3 or 4 small dates, pitted**

**1 teaspoon coconut oil**

**1 teaspoon maple syrup**

**⅛ teaspoon ground cinnamon**

**⅛ teaspoon vanilla extract**

**⅛ teaspoon sea salt**

1. Preheat the oven to 400°F.

2. Core each apple, but leave the bottom intact to form a cup. Place each apple on a 8-inch square of aluminum foil.

3. In a high-speed blender or food processor, combine the oats, shredded coconut, dates, coconut oil, maple syrup, cinnamon, vanilla, and salt and blend until well combined.

4. Stuff each apple with approximately 2 tablespoons of the oat mixture.

5. Wrap the foil around each apple, leaving a bit of the top exposed, and place the apples on a baking sheet. Bake for 20 to 25 minutes, until the apples are soft and the filling is golden.

**MAKE IT EASIER:** If it's difficult to core the apple while retaining its shape, simply slice it, layer the slices in the foil, and top with the crumble. Wrap with the foil similarly to expose only the crumble to keep the apple inside moist.

**Per Serving (1 baked apple)**: Calories: 162; Fat: 5g; Protein: 1g; Carbohydrates: 32g; Fiber: 6g; Sodium: 75mg; Iron: 1mg

# PB Frosting

MAKES ¾ CUP
**PREP TIME:** 5 minutes

Nope, this isn't really frosting, but it'll definitely satisfy your sweet tooth. Made with chickpeas and peanut butter, its creamy sweetness—without excess fats and sugars—is provided by maple syrup (or dates). Spread it on whole-grain toast or dip apple slices in it.

**¾ cup canned low-sodium chickpeas, drained (liquid reserved) and rinsed**

**2 tablespoons peanut butter or all-natural nut butter of your choice**

**2 tablespoons maple syrup, or 8 small dates, pitted**

**⅛ teaspoon sea salt**

**⅛ teaspoon vanilla extract**

**⅛ teaspoon ground cinnamon**

In a high-speed blender, combine the chickpeas, peanut butter, maple syrup, salt, vanilla, and cinnamon. Blend until smooth and creamy.

**SUBSTITUTION TIP:** If you replace the chickpeas with black beans and add 1 to 2 tablespoons unsweetened carob powder or cocoa powder, you'll have a delicious chocolate frosting.

**Per Serving (2 tablespoons)**: Calories: 76; Fat: 3g; Protein: 2g; Carbohydrates: 10g; Fiber: 2g; Sodium: 90mg; Iron: 0mg

# Banana-Cashew Nice Cream

**SERVES 6**

**PREP TIME:** 3 minutes (plus overnight soaking)

Made with just a few basic ingredients, this "nice cream" is basically fruit and nuts, so you get the benefit of two food groups in one treat.

4 ripe medium bananas, sliced and frozen

1 cup cashews, soaked in 2 cups water overnight, then drained

½ cup water

1 tablespoon unsweetened carob powder, ground cinnamon, or unsweetened cocoa powder

½ teaspoon vanilla extract

⅛ teaspoon sea salt

In a high-speed blender, combine the frozen bananas, cashews, water, carob powder, vanilla, and salt. Blend until smooth and creamy, then serve immediately.

**SUBSTITUTION TIP:** Try this with nut butter instead. Simply replace the cashews with 3 tablespoons of your choice of nut butter.

Per Serving (about ½ cup): Calories: 200; Fat: 10g; Protein: 5g; Carbohydrates: 25g; Fiber: 3g; Sodium: 53mg; Iron: 2mg

# Carrot Cake Cookies with Cashew Cream Frosting

**MAKES 12 COOKIES**

**PREP TIME:** 5 to 7 minutes (plus overnight soaking)
**COOK TIME:** 12 minutes

These cookies are a perfect treat for holidays, or any time you like. The cashews serve as the base for the frosting. Be sure to soak them the night before you plan to prepare this recipe so you won't have to wait for the nuts to soften the next day.

**FOR THE CARROT CAKE COOKIES**

10 small dates, pitted

¼ cup cashew butter

¼ cup unsweetened finely shredded coconut

¼ cup almond meal

1 medium egg

1 tablespoon coconut oil

¼ teaspoon vanilla extract

¼ teaspoon ground cinnamon

⅛ teaspoon sea salt

¾ cup rolled oats

¼ cup brown rice flour

½ teaspoon baking soda

¼ cup golden raisins

**To make the carrot cake cookies**

1. Preheat the oven to 375°F. Line a baking sheet with parchment paper.

2. In a food processor, combine the dates, cashew butter, shredded coconut, almond meal, egg, coconut oil, vanilla, cinnamon, and salt. Blend until smooth and well combined.

3. In a medium bowl, combine the oats, brown rice flour, and baking soda. Add the wet ingredients and stir to combine well.

4. Fold in the raisins, walnuts, and carrot.

5. Scoop the mixture into 1½-inch balls and place them on the prepared baking sheet, spacing them evenly. Bake for 12 minutes, or until a toothpick inserted into the center of a cookie comes out clean. Let cool completely.

3 tablespoons
chopped walnuts

2 tablespoons
shredded carrot

**FOR THE CASHEW
CREAM FROSTING**

1 cup cashews,
soaked in water
overnight,
then drained

8 small dates, pitted

½ cup water

¼ cup unsweetened
shredded coconut

1 to 2 teaspoons
freshly squeezed
lemon juice
(optional)

¼ teaspoon
vanilla extract

⅛ teaspoon sea salt

To make the cashew cream frosting

6. In a high-speed blender, combine the cashews, dates, water, shredded coconut, lemon juice (if using), vanilla, and salt. Blend until well combined, with date specks sprinkled throughout.

7. Frost each cookie with about 1 rounded teaspoon of the cashew cream frosting.

INGREDIENT SWAP: You can replace the egg by stirring together 1 tablespoon flax meal and 2 tablespoons water and letting the mixture stand until gelled and thickened. Use the flax mixture where the egg is called for in the recipe.

Per Serving (1 cookie): Calories: 166; Fat: 9g; Protein: 4g; Carbohydrates: 20g; Fiber: 3g; Sodium: 100mg; Iron: 1mg

# Cashew Date Oat Bites

MAKES 20 BITES
**PREP TIME:** 3 minutes / **COOK TIME:** 10 minutes

These oat bites are perfect for breakfast, as a snack, or any time you'd like a sweet and satisfying option.

**Nonstick cooking spray**

**¾ cup rolled oats**

**8 small dates, pitted**

**¼ cup unsweetened coconut flakes (optional)**

**¼ cup cashew butter**

**1 teaspoon ground cinnamon**

**½ teaspoon vanilla extract**

**3 to 4 tablespoons water**

**½ cup raisins**

1. Preheat the oven to 350°F. Lightly grease a baking sheet with cooking spray.

2. In a food processor, combine the oats, dates, coconut flakes (if using), cashew butter, cinnamon, and vanilla. Process until the mixture resembles coarse crumbs.

3. Add the water 1 tablespoon at a time, until a dough forms and holds together well. Transfer the mixture to a bowl and mix in the raisins until evenly distributed throughout the dough.

4. Using a mini scoop or rounded teaspoon, scoop small balls of the mixture onto the prepared baking sheet, spacing them evenly.

5. Bake for 10 minutes, or until just browned. Do not overcook.

**SUBSTITUTION TIP:** Use chocolate chips instead of raisins.

**MAKE IT EASIER:** For an energy bite treat, simply refrigerate the unbaked bites on the baking sheet for 30 minutes, then transfer to an airtight container and refrigerate for up to 2 weeks or freeze for up to 2 months.

**Per Serving (2 bites):** Calories: 113; Fat: 5g; Protein: 2g; Carbohydrates: 17g; Fiber: 2g; Sodium: 4mg; Iron: 1mg

# Vegan Waldorf Salad

SERVES 6

**PREP TIME:** 5 minutes

This creamy fruit salad is as satisfying as it is sweet. This vegan version uses homemade vegan mayo and no added sugars, but you won't miss a thing.

5 tablespoons Creamy Vegan Mayonnaise (see page 74)

1 tablespoon freshly squeezed lemon juice

2 apples, cored and chopped

1 cup halved seedless grapes

1 cup sliced celery

½ cup hulled pumpkin seeds

2 small dates, pitted and finely chopped, or 1 tablespoon raisins

3 cups chopped romaine lettuce

1. In a medium bowl, mix the mayonnaise and lemon juice.

2. Add the apples, grapes, celery, pumpkin seeds, and dates and toss to coat well.

3. Place ½ cup of the lettuce on each serving plate, divide the fruit mixture evenly among them, and serve.

**SUBSTITUTION TIP:** Swap out the pumpkin seeds for an equal amount of chopped walnuts. These nuts offer heart-healthy omega-3s in addition to vitamin E, vitamin $B_6$, and phosphorus.

**Per Serving**: Calories: 199; Fat: 14g; Protein: 4g; Carbohydrates: 18g; Fiber: 3g; Sodium: 31mg; Iron: 1mg

# The Ultimate Alkaline Food Guide

The Ultimate Alkaline Food Guide is a tool to support your health journey. Foods are ranked according to their levels of alkalinity or acidity. Any food within the alkaline range is fine to consume. When choosing foods in the acid range, aim for those that are low to medium in acidic value. That doesn't mean you can't enjoy a more highly acidic food every once in a while; just stick to the 80/20 rule.

This is a plant-driven guide, focusing on plenty of fruits and vegetables, including beans and legumes, and whole-grain foods (low to mildly acidic, but still very healthy for you). There is a wide variety of foods to choose from, plus flexibility as per the spectrum of alkalinity and acidity provided. Be sure to limit highly processed foods, animal proteins, and dairy to special occasions.

# Acid-Alkaline Ratings Charts

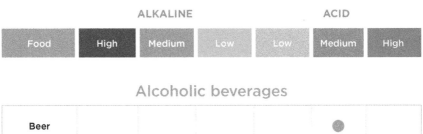

| Food | ALKALINE | | | ACID | | |
|------|------|--------|-----|-----|--------|------|
| | High | Medium | Low | Low | Medium | High |

## Alcoholic beverages

| Food | High | Medium | Low | Low | Medium | High |
|------|------|--------|-----|-----|--------|------|
| Beer | | | | | ● | |
| Wine, red | | | | | ● | |

## Vinegar And Oil

| Food | High | Medium | Low | Low | Medium | High |
|------|------|--------|-----|-----|--------|------|
| Apple cider vinegar | ● | | | | | |
| Avocado oil | | ● | | | | |
| Balsamic vinegar | | | | ● | | |
| Coconut oil | | ● | | | | |
| Olive oil | | ● | | | | |

## Beans and Legumes

| Food | High | Medium | Low | Low | Medium | High |
|------|------|--------|-----|-----|--------|------|
| Adzuki beans | | | ● | | | |
| Baked beans, vegetarian | | | ● | | | |
| Black beans | | | ● | | | |

| Food | ALKALINE | | | ACID | | |
|------|----------|--------|-----|-----|--------|------|
|      | High | Medium | Low | Low | Medium | High |

## Beans and Legumes *continued*

| Food | High | Medium | Low | Low | Medium | High |
|------|------|--------|-----|-----|--------|------|
| Chickpeas | | | | ● | | |
| Edamame | | | ● | | | |
| Great northern beans | | | | ● | | |
| Kidney beans | | | | ● | | |
| Lentils | ● | | | | | |
| Lima beans | | | | ● | | |
| Navy beans | | | | ● | | |
| Peanuts | | | | | ● | |
| Peas, fresh green | | | | ● | | |
| Peas, split green and yellow | | | | ● | | |
| Pinto beans | | | | ● | | |
| Snow peas | | | ● | | | |
| Soybeans | | | | | | ● |
| String beans | | | | ● | | |
| Tofu | | | | ● | | |

| | ALKALINE | | | ACID | | |
|---|---|---|---|---|---|---|
| Food | High | Medium | Low | Low | Medium | High |

## Beef/Pork

| | High | Medium | Low | Low | Medium | High |
|---|---|---|---|---|---|---|
| Bacon | | | | | | ● |
| Frankfurters | | | | | | ● |
| Hamburgers | | | | | | ● |
| Steak (steaks, roasts, etc.) | | | | | | ● |

## Berries

| | High | Medium | Low | Low | Medium | High |
|---|---|---|---|---|---|---|
| Blackberries | ● | | | | | |
| Blueberries | | ● | | | | |
| Cherries | | ● | | | | |
| Raspberries | ● | | | | | |
| Strawberries | ● | | | | | |

## Beverages

| | High | Medium | Low | Low | Medium | High |
|---|---|---|---|---|---|---|
| Apple juice, unsweetened | | | ● | | | |
| Carrot juice | | | | ● | | |
| Coconut milk, can or carton | | ● | | | | |

| Food | High | Medium | Low | Low | Medium | High |
|------|------|--------|-----|-----|--------|------|

## Beverages *continued*

| Food | High | Medium | Low | Low | Medium | High |
|------|------|--------|-----|-----|--------|------|
| Coffee, regular | | | | | ● | |
| Coffee, espresso | | | | | | ● |
| Cola | | | | | | ● |
| Grape juice | | | ● | | | |
| Grapefruit juice | | ● | | | | |
| Milk, 1% fat | | | | ● | | |
| Milk, nonfat | | | | ● | | |
| Milk, almond unsweetened | | | ● | | | |
| Milk, rice | | | | | ● | |
| Milk, soy | | | | ● | | |
| Orange juice | | | ● | | | |
| Tea, black | | | | ● | | |
| Tea, green | | | ● | | | |
| Tea, herbal | | | ● | | | |

| Food | ALKALINE | | | ACID | | |
|------|----------|--------|-----|-----|--------|------|
|  | High | Medium | Low | Low | Medium | High |

## Bread

| Food | High | Medium | Low | Low | Medium | High |
|------|------|--------|-----|-----|--------|------|
| Bagel, plain | | | | | | ● |
| English muffins | | | | | | ● |
| Matzo, white flour | | | | | | ● |
| Pita, whole wheat flour | | | | | ● | |
| Pumpernickel | | | | | ● | |
| 100% rye bread | | | | | ● | |
| Tortillas, corn | | | | | ● | |
| Tortillas, white flour | | | | | | ● |
| Whole wheat bread | | | | | ● | |

## Dairy products

| Food | High | Medium | Low | Low | Medium | High |
|------|------|--------|-----|-----|--------|------|
| American cheese | | | | | | ● |
| Cheddar cheese | | | | | | ● |
| Cottage cheese | | | | | ● | |

| Food | ALKALINE | | | ACID | | |
| | High | Medium | Low | Low | Medium | High |
|---|---|---|---|---|---|---|

## Dairy products *continued*

| Food | High | Medium | Low | Low | Medium | High |
|---|---|---|---|---|---|---|
| Cream cheese | | | | | ● | |
| Egg, white only | | | | ● | | |
| Egg, whole | | | | ● | | |
| Mozzarella cheese | | | | | | ● |
| Swiss cheese | | | | | | ● |

## Fish

| Food | High | Medium | Low | Low | Medium | High |
|---|---|---|---|---|---|---|
| Bass | | | | | ● | |
| Catfish | | | | | ● | |
| Crab | | | | | ● | |
| Flounder | | | | | ● | |
| Grouper | | | | | ● | |
| Salmon | | | | | ● | |
| Shrimp | | | | | | ● |
| Tuna | | | | | ● | |

| Food | ALKALINE | | | ACID | | |
|------|----------|--------|-----|-----|--------|------|
| | High | Medium | Low | Low | Medium | High |

## Flours

| Food | High | Medium | Low | Low | Medium | High |
|------|------|--------|-----|-----|--------|------|
| Almond flour | | ● | | | | |
| Amaranth flour | | | ● | | | |
| Barley flour | | | | ● | | |
| Buckwheat flour | | | ● | | | |
| Millet flour | | | ● | | | |
| Oat flour | | ● | | | | |
| Rice flour, brown | | | ● | | | |
| Wheat flour, white | | | | | | ● |
| Wheat flour, whole | | | | | ● | |

## Grains

| Food | High | Medium | Low | Low | Medium | High |
|------|------|--------|-----|-----|--------|------|
| Barley, whole grain | | | | | ● | |
| Bulgur wheat | | | | | ● | |
| Corn | | | | | ● | |
| Cornmeal | | | | | ● | |

| Food | ALKALINE | | | ACID | | |
|------|----------|--------|-----|-----|--------|------|
| | High | Medium | Low | Low | Medium | High |

## Grains *continued*

| Food | High | Medium | Low | Low | Medium | High |
|------|------|--------|-----|-----|--------|------|
| Freekeh | | | | ● | | |
| Kasha (buckwheat groats) | | | | ● | | |
| Millet | | | | ● | | |
| Oat bran | | | | | ● | |
| Polenta | | | | | ● | |
| Quinoa | | | ● | | | |
| Rice, brown | | | | ● | | |
| Rice, white | | | | | ● | |
| Rice, wild | | | ● | | | |
| Wheat, unrefined | | | | ● | | |

## Fruits

| Food | High | Medium | Low | Low | Medium | High |
|------|------|--------|-----|-----|--------|------|
| Apple | | ● | | | | |
| Apricot | | ● | | | | |
| Avocado | | ● | | | | |

| Food | ALKALINE | | | ACID | | |
| --- | --- | --- | --- | --- | --- | --- |
| | High | Medium | Low | Low | Medium | High |
| **Fruits** *continued* | | | | | | |
| Banana | | ● | | | | |
| Cantaloupe | ● | | | | | |
| Coconuts | | | ● | | | |
| Date | | | | ● | | |
| Fig | | | | ● | | |
| Grapefruit | | ● | | | | |
| Grapes | | ● | | | | |
| Kiwi fruit | ● | | | | | |
| Lemon | | ● | | | | |
| Mango | ● | | | | | |
| Orange | | ● | | | | |
| Papaya | ● | | | | | |
| Peach | | ● | | | | |
| Pineapple | ● | | | | | |
| Plum | | | | ● | | |

| Food | ALKALINE | | | ACID | | |
| | High | Medium | Low | Low | Medium | High |
|------|------|--------|-----|-----|--------|------|

## Fruits *continued*

| Food | High | Medium | Low | Low | Medium | High |
|------|------|--------|-----|-----|--------|------|
| Pomegranate | | | | | ● | |
| Tomato | | | | ● | | |
| Watermelon | ● | | | | | |

## Herbs and spices

| Food | High | Medium | Low | Low | Medium | High |
|------|------|--------|-----|-----|--------|------|
| Basil | | ● | | | | |
| Cilantro | | ● | | | | |
| Cinnamon | | ● | | | | |
| Cumin | | ● | | | | |
| Curry | | | | ● | | |
| Dill | | ● | | | | |
| Ginger root | ● | | | | | |
| Oregano | | ● | | | | |
| Paprika | ● | | | | | |
| Pepper - black | | ● | | | | |
| Salt | | | | | | ● |

| Food | ALKALINE | | | ACID | | |
|------|----------|--------|-----|-----|--------|------|
| | High | Medium | Low | Low | Medium | High |

## Nut Butters

| Food | High | Medium | Low | Low | Medium | High |
|------|------|--------|-----|-----|--------|------|
| Almond butter | | | ● | | | |
| Cashew butter | ● | | | | | |
| Peanut butter | | | | | ● | |

## Nuts and Seeds

| Food | High | Medium | Low | Low | Medium | High |
|------|------|--------|-----|-----|--------|------|
| Almonds | | | ● | | | |
| Cashews | ● | | | | | |
| Chia seeds | | | ● | | | |
| Flaxseed | | | ● | | | |
| Hazelnuts | | | | | | ● |
| Hemp seeds | | | ● | | | |
| Macadamia nuts | | | ● | | | |
| Peanuts | | | | | ● | |
| Pecans | | | | | ● | |
| Pistachio nuts | | | | | ● | |

| Food | ALKALINE | | | ACID | | |
|---|---|---|---|---|---|---|
| | High | Medium | Low | Low | Medium | High |

## Nuts and Seeds *continued*

| Food | High | Medium | Low | Low | Medium | High |
|---|---|---|---|---|---|---|
| Pumpkin seeds | ● | | | | | |
| Sunflower seeds | | | ● | | | |
| Walnuts | | | | | | ● |

## Pasta

| Food | High | Medium | Low | Low | Medium | High |
|---|---|---|---|---|---|---|
| Spaghetti, rye | | | | | ● | |
| Spaghetti, white flour | | | | | | ● |
| Spaghetti, whole wheat flour | | | | | ● | |

## Poultry

| Food | High | Medium | Low | Low | Medium | High |
|---|---|---|---|---|---|---|
| Chicken | | | | | ● | |
| Duck | | | | | ● | |
| Turkey | | | | | ● | |

| Food | ALKALINE | | | ACID | | |
|------|----------|--------|-----|-----|--------|------|
| | High | Medium | Low | Low | Medium | High |

## Root vegetables

| Food | High | Medium | Low | Low | Medium | High |
|------|------|--------|-----|-----|--------|------|
| Cassava | | ● | | | | |
| Taro | | ● | | | | |
| Yucca | | ● | | | | |
| Beets | | ● | | | | |

## Sweeteners

| Food | High | Medium | Low | Low | Medium | High |
|------|------|--------|-----|-----|--------|------|
| Agave nectar | | ● | | | | |
| Artificial, aspartame | | | | | ● | |
| Artificial, saccharin | | | | | ● | |
| Corn syrup | | | | | | ● |
| Honey | | | | ● | | |
| Maple syrup | | | | ● | | |
| Molasses | | ● | | | | |
| Stevia | | | | ● | | |
| Sugar, brown | | | | | | ● |
| Sugar, white | | | | | | ● |

| Food | High | Medium | Low | Low | Medium | High |
|---|---|---|---|---|---|---|

## Vegetables

| Food | High (Alk) | Medium (Alk) | Low (Alk) | Low (Acid) | Medium (Acid) | High (Acid) |
|---|---|---|---|---|---|---|
| Artichokes | | ● | | | | |
| Asparagus | ● | | | | | |
| Bell peppers | | ● | | | | |
| Broccoli | | ● | | | | |
| Brussels sprouts | | | ● | | | |
| Cabbage | | ● | | | | |
| Carrots, conventional | | | | ● | | |
| Carrots, organic | | | ● | | | |
| Cauliflower | | ● | | | | |
| Celery | | ● | | | | |
| Chard, Swiss | | | | ● | | |
| Corn | | | | | ● | |
| Cucumbers | | | ● | | | |
| Eggplant | | ● | | | | |
| Kale | ● | | | | | |

| | ALKALINE | | | ACID | | |
|---|---|---|---|---|---|---|
| Food | High | Medium | Low | Low | Medium | High |

## Vegetables *continued*

| | High | Medium | Low | Low | Medium | High |
|---|---|---|---|---|---|---|
| Leeks | | ● | | | | |
| Lettuce, arugula | | ● | | | | |
| Lettuce, iceberg | | ● | | | | |
| Lettuce, red leaf | | ● | | | | |
| Lettuce, rocket | | ● | | | | |
| Lettuce, romaine | | ● | | | | |
| Mushrooms | | | ● | | | |
| Mustard greens | ● | | | | | |
| Okra | | ● | | | | |
| Onions | ● | | | | | |
| Parsnips | ● | | | | | |
| Potato, white | | ● | | | | |
| Potato, sweet | ● | | | | | |
| Radishes | ● | | | | | |
| Scallions | | ● | | | | |

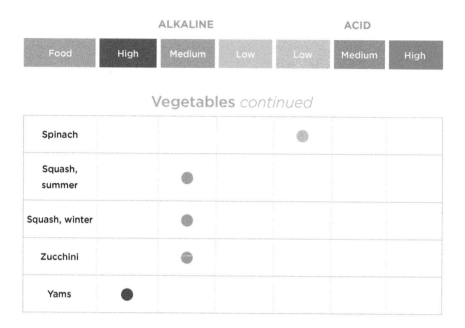

| Food | ALKALINE High | ALKALINE Medium | ALKALINE Low | ACID Low | ACID Medium | ACID High |
|------|------|------|------|------|------|------|

## Vegetables *continued*

| Food | High | Medium | Low | Low | Medium | High |
|------|------|--------|-----|-----|--------|------|
| Spinach | | | | ● | | |
| Squash, summer | | ● | | | | |
| Squash, winter | | ● | | | | |
| Zucchini | | ● | | | | |
| Yams | ● | | | | | |

## Water

| Food | High | Medium | Low | Low | Medium | High |
|------|------|--------|-----|-----|--------|------|
| Bottled mineral, Evian | | | ● | | | |
| Bottled mineral, Fiji | | | ● | | | |
| Tap, chlorinated | | | | | ● | |

## Miscellaneous

| Food | High | Medium | Low | Low | Medium | High |
|------|------|--------|-----|-----|--------|------|
| Baking chocolate | | | | | | ● |
| Barbeque sauce | | | | | ● | |
| Brownies | | | | | | ● |
| Butter | | | | ● | | |

| Food | High | Medium | Low | Low | Medium | High |
|------|------|--------|-----|-----|--------|------|

## Miscellaneous *continued*

| Food | High | Medium | Low | Low | Medium | High |
|------|------|--------|-----|-----|--------|------|
| Burrito, with beef | | | | | | ● |
| Burrito, with chicken | | | | | | ● |
| Cheesecake | | | | | | ● |
| Croutons | | | | | | ● |
| Donuts | | | | | | ● |
| Horseradish | ● | | | | | |
| Hummus | | | | ● | | |
| Ketchup | | | | | ● | |
| Mayonnaise | | | | ● | | |
| Miso | ● | | | | | |
| Mustard | | | | | ● | |
| Pizza | | | | | | ● |
| Popcorn | | | | | ● | |
| Potato chips | | | | | | ● |
| Tortilla chips | | | | | | ● |

# Measurement Conversions

| | US STANDARD | US STANDARD (OUNCES) | METRIC (APPROXIMATE) |
|---|---|---|---|
| **VOLUME EQUIVALENTS (LIQUID)** | 2 tablespoons | 1 fl. oz. | 30 mL |
| | ¼ cup | 2 fl. oz. | 60 mL |
| | ½ cup | 4 fl. oz. | 120 mL |
| | 1 cup | 8 fl. oz. | 240 mL |
| | 1½ cups | 12 fl. oz. | 355 mL |
| | 2 cups or 1 pint | 16 fl. oz. | 475 mL |
| | 4 cups or 1 quart | 32 fl. oz. | 1 L |
| | 1 gallon | 128 fl. oz. | 4 L |
| **VOLUME EQUIVALENTS (DRY)** | ⅛ teaspoon | | 0.5 mL |
| | ¼ teaspoon | | 1 mL |
| | ½ teaspoon | | 2 mL |
| | ¾ teaspoon | | 4 mL |
| | 1 teaspoon | | 5 mL |
| | 1 tablespoon | | 15 mL |
| | ¼ cup | | 59 mL |
| | ⅓ cup | | 79 mL |
| | ½ cup | | 118 mL |
| | ⅔ cup | | 156 mL |
| | ¾ cup | | 177 mL |
| | 1 cup | | 235 mL |
| | 2 cups or 1 pint | | 475 mL |
| | 3 cups | | 700 mL |
| | 4 cups or 1 quart | | 1 L |
| | ½ gallon | | 2 L |
| | 1 gallon | | 4 L |
| **WEIGHT EQUIVALENTS** | ½ ounce | | 15 g |
| | 1 ounce | | 30 g |
| | 2 ounces | | 60 g |
| | 4 ounces | | 115 g |
| | 8 ounces | | 225 g |
| | 12 ounces | | 340 g |
| | 16 ounces or 1 pound | | 455 g |

|  | FAHRENHEIT (F) | CELSIUS (C) (APPROXIMATE) |
|---|---|---|
| OVEN TEMPERATURES | 250°F | 120°C |
|  | 300°F | 150°C |
|  | 325°F | 180°C |
|  | 375°F | 190°C |
|  | 400°F | 200°C |
|  | 425°F | 220°C |
|  | 450°F | 230°C |

# References

American Institute for Cancer Research. "Another Cancer and Diet Claim: The Alkaline Diet." Accessed February 26, 2020. https://www.aicr.org/resources/blog/another-cancer-and-diet-claim-the-alkaline-diet/.

American Institute for Cancer Research. "Eat a Diet Rich in Whole Grains, Vegetables, Fruits, and Beans." Accessed March 2, 2020. https://www.aicr.org/cancer-prevention/recommendations/eat-a-diet-rich-in-whole-grains-vegetables-fruits-and-beans/.

Aviv, Jonathan. "Why the Alkaline Ash Diet Is Not Healthy for Acid Reflux Sufferers." Accessed March 3, 2020. https://www.acidwatcher.com/index.php/blog/entry/why-the-alkaline-ash-diet-is-not-healthy-for-acid-reflux-sufferers.

Clarrett, Danisa M., and Christine Hachem. "Gastroesophageal Reflux Disease (GERD)." *Missouri Medicine* 115, no. 3 (2018): 214–18.

Engberink, Marielle F., Stephan J. L. Bakker, Elizabeth J. Brink, Marleen A. Van Baak, Frank Ja Van Rooij, Albert Hofman, Jacqueline C. M. Witteman, and Johanna M. Geleijnse. "Dietary Acid Load and Risk of Hypertension: the Rotterdam Study." *American Journal of Clinical Nutrition* 95, no. 6 (February 2012): 1438–44. doi.org/10.3945/ajcn.111.022343.

Farhangi, Mahdieh Abbasalizad, Leila Nikniaz, and Zeinab Nikniaz. "Higher Dietary Acid Load Potentially Increases Serum Triglyceride and Obesity Prevalence in Adults: An Updated Systematic Review and Meta-Analysis." *PLOS ONE* 14, no. 5 (September 2019). doi.org/10.1371/journal.pone.0216547.

Fenton, Tanis R., Michael Eliasziw, Andrew W. Lyon, Suzanne C. Tough, and David A. Hanley. "Meta-Analysis of the Quantity of Calcium Excretion Associated with the Net Acid Excretion of the Modern Diet under the Acid-Ash Diet Hypothesis." *American Journal of Clinical Nutrition* 88, no. 4 (January 2008): 1159–66. doi.org/10.1093/ajcn/88.4.1159.

Fenton, Tanis R., Andrew W. Lyon, Michael Eliasziw, Suzanne C. Tough, and David A. Hanley. "Meta-Analysis of the Effect of the Acid-Ash Hypothesis of Osteoporosis on Calcium Balance." *Journal of Bone and Mineral Research* 24, no. 11 (2009): 1835–40. doi.org/10.1359/jbmr.090515.

Fenton, Tanis R., Suzanne C. Tough, Andrew W. Lyon, Misha Eliasziw, and David A. Hanley. "Causal Assessment of Dietary Acid Load and Bone Disease: A Systematic Review & Meta-Analysis Applying Hills Epidemiologic Criteria for Causality." *Nutrition Journal* 10, no. 1 (2011). doi.org/10.1186/1475-2891-10-41.

Fenton, Tanis R., and Tian Huang. "Systematic Review of the Association Between Dietary Acid Load, Alkaline Water, and Cancer." *BMJ Open* 6, no. 6 (2016). doi.org/10.1136/bmjopen-2015-010438.

Haddy, Francis J., Paul M. Vanhoutte, and Michel Feletou. "Role of Potassium in Regulating Blood Flow and Blood Pressure." *American Journal of Physiology-Regulatory, Integrative and Comparative Physiology* 290, no. 3 (2006). doi.org/10.1152/ajpregu.00491.2005.

Hever, Julieanna, and Raymond J. Cronise. "Plant-Based Nutrition for Healthcare Professionals: Implementing Diet as a Primary Modality in the Prevention and Treatment of Chronic Disease." *Journal of Geriatric Cardiology: JGC* 14, no. 5 (2017): 355–68. doi:10.11909/j.issn.1671-5411.2017.05.012.

International Osteoporosis Foundation. "Smoking Is a Real Danger to Your Bone Health." Accessed March 3, 2020. https://www.iofbonehealth.org/news/smoking-real-danger-your-bone-health.

Johnson, Mary Ann. "If High Folic Acid Aggravates Vitamin B12 Deficiency What Should Be Done About It?" *Nutrition Reviews* 65, no. 10 (2008): 451–58. doi.org/10.1111/j.1753-4887.2007.tb00270.x.

Kovesdy, Csaba P. "Metabolic Acidosis and Progression of Chronic Kidney Disease." *Metabolic Acidosis* (2016): 131–43. doi.org/10.1007/978-1-4939-3463-8_13.

Kramer, Holly. "Diet and Chronic Kidney Disease." *Advances in Nutrition* 10, Supplement 4 (January 2019). doi.org/10.1093/advances/nmz011.

Krupp, Danika, Jonas Esche, Gert Mensink, Stefanie Klenow, Michael Thamm, and Thomas Remer. "Dietary Acid Load and Potassium Intake Associate with Blood Pressure and Hypertension Prevalence in a Representative Sample of the German Adult Population." *Nutrients* 10, no. 1 (2018): 103. doi.org/10.3390/nu10010103.

Law, M. R., and A. K. Hackshaw. "A Meta-Analysis of Cigarette Smoking, Bone Mineral Density and Risk of Hip Fracture: Recognition of a Major Effect." *BMJ* 315, no. 7112 (April 1997): 841–46. doi.org/10.1136/bmj.315.7112.841.

Lips, P., and N. M. Van Schoor. "The Effect of Vitamin D on Bone and Osteoporosis." *Best Practice & Research Clinical Endocrinology & Metabolism* 25, no. 4 (August 2011): 585–91. doi: 10.1016/j.beem.2011.05.002.

London: National Institute for Health and Care Excellence (UK) "Eating Disorders: Recognition and Treatment." Accessed March 3, 2020. https://www.nice.org.uk/guidance/ng69/resources/eating-disorders-recognition-and-treatment-pdf-1837582159813.

Makki, Kassem, Edward C. Deehan, Jens Walter, and Fredrik Bäckhed. "The Impact of Dietary Fiber on Gut Microbiota in Host Health and Disease." *Cell Host & Microbe* 23, no. 6 (2018): 705–15. doi.org/10.1016/j.chom.2018.05.012.

Mayo Clinic. Mayo Foundation for Medical Education and Research. "Low Potassium (Hypokalemia) Causes." Accessed March 2, 2020. https://www.mayoclinic.org/symptoms/low-potassium/basics/causes/sym-20050632.

Melamed, Peter, and Felix Melamed Felix. "Chronic Metabolic Acidosis Destroys Pancreas." *Journal of the Pancreas* 15, no. 6 (November 2014): 541–632.

Merck Manuals Consumer Version. Merck Manuals. "Alkalosis - Hormonal and Metabolic Disorders." Accessed March 3, 2020. https://www.merckmanuals.com/home/hormonal-and-metabolic-disorders/acid-base-balance/alkalosis.

National Institutes of Health. U.S. Department of Health and Human Services. "Smoking and Bone Health." Accessed

March 3, 2020. https://www.bones.nih.gov/health-info/bone
/osteoporosis/conditions-behaviors/bone-smoking.

National Osteoporosis Foundation. "Prevention and Healthy Living."
Accessed March 3, 2020. https://www.nof.org/preventing-fractures
/prevention/prevention-and-healthy-living/.

Nettleton, J. A. "Omega-3 Fatty Acids. Comparison of Plant and Seafood Sources in Human Nutrition." *Journal of the American Dietetic
Association* 91, no. 3 (March 1991): 331–37. PubMed PMID: 1825498.

Nicoll, Rachel, and John McLaren Howard. "The Acid–Ash Hypothesis Revisited: A Reassessment of the Impact of Dietary Acidity on
Bone." *Journal of Bone and Mineral Metabolism* 32, no. 5 (2014):
469–75. doi.org/10.1007/s00774-014-0571-0.

Pan, Li-Long, Jiahong Li, Muhammad Shamoon, Madhav Bhatia,
and Jia Sun. "Corrigendum: Recent Advances on Nutrition in
Treatment of Acute Pancreatitis." *Frontiers in Immunology* 9 (2018).
doi.org/10.3389/fimmu.2018.00849.

Rizzo, Gianluca, Antonio Laganà, Agnese Rapisarda, Gioacchina
La Ferrera, Massimo Buscema, Paola Rossetti, Angela Nigro, et al.
"Vitamin B12 among Vegetarians: Status, Assessment and Supple-
mentation." *Nutrients* 8, no. 12 (2016): 767. doi.org/10.3390/nu8120767.

Scialla, Julia J., and Cheryl A. M. Anderson. "Dietary Acid Load:
A Novel Nutritional Target in Chronic Kidney Disease?" *Advances
in Chronic Kidney Disease* 20, no. 2 (2013): 141–49. doi.org/10.1053
/j.ackd.2012.11.001.

Singh, R. K., H. W. Chang, D. Yan, K. M. Lee, D. Ucmak, K. Wong,
M. Abrouk, B. Farahnik, M. Nakamura, T. H. Zhu, T. Bhutani, and
W. Liao. "Influence of Diet on the Gut Microbiome and Implications
for Human Health." *Journal of Translational Medicine* 15, no. 73
(April 2017). doi.org/10.1186/s12967-017-1175-y.

Uribarri, Jaime, and Mona S. Calvo. "Dietary Phosphorus Excess:
A Risk Factor in Chronic Bone, Kidney, and Cardiovascular Disease?"
*Advances in Nutrition* 4, no. 5 (January 2013): 542–44.
doi.org/10.3945/an.113.004234.

# Index

# Acknowledgments

I'd like to acknowledge my family, my friends, and all of those who've supported me along the way. To my loving husband, JP, for supporting my career and endeavors such as this book. Hugs and kisses to my twin daughters, Ailish and Julia, for being enthusiastic "taste testers," and for keeping themselves content and occupied during my countless hours on my laptop. My girls assisted in tasks such as chopping and mixing during some of my final recipe trials. And to my friends Briana and Bridie for cheering me on and keeping me sane. I'd also like to thank my mom for always believing in me (I know my dad would be smiling in heaven). And a huge thank-you to my editor, Justin Hartung, for his encouragement, positive feedback, and guidance throughout this project. He gave me the space to be creative while keeping me on point.

# About the Author

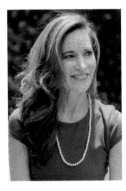

**Lauren O'Connor** is a registered dietitian/nutritionist and yoga instructor. She offers nutritional counseling and consulting services for individuals and companies nationwide. She received her master's degree in nutritional sciences from California State University, Los Angeles, and is a member of the Academy of Nutrition and Dietetics (AND) and Food & Culinary Professionals (FCP). As a recipe developer and credentialed health advocate, she is sought out for her expert opinion in various national media outlets, including print, TV, and radio.

O'Connor promotes whole food choices and plant-based nutrition, tailoring plans and recipes to best suit her clients' needs. With a specialty in GERD management, she promotes dietary and lifestyle practices to improve health outcomes for those with acid reflux concerns.

CPSIA information can be obtained
at www.ICGtesting.com
Printed in the USA
BVHW092117051121
620893BV00004B/4